Dr. Joe Bell

Dr. Joe Bell

Model for Sherlock Holmes

Ely Liebow

Popular Press

Popular Press
An imprint of the University of Wisconsin Press
1930 Monroe Street
Madison, Wisconsin 53711

3 Henrietta Street
London WC2E 8LU, England

www.wisc.edu\wisconsinpress

Originally published by Bowling Green University Popular Press
Copyright © 1982
Bowling Green University Popular Press

Printed in the United States of America

Library of Congress Catalog Card No.: 81-85520

ISBN: 0-87972-197-9 Clothbound
       0-87972-198-7 Paperback

To
Phoebe
(Joe Bell's kind of nurse)
and
"The Girls"

For whom it was a pleasure and privilege
to read the Canon—at least twice over.

Illustrations

Contents

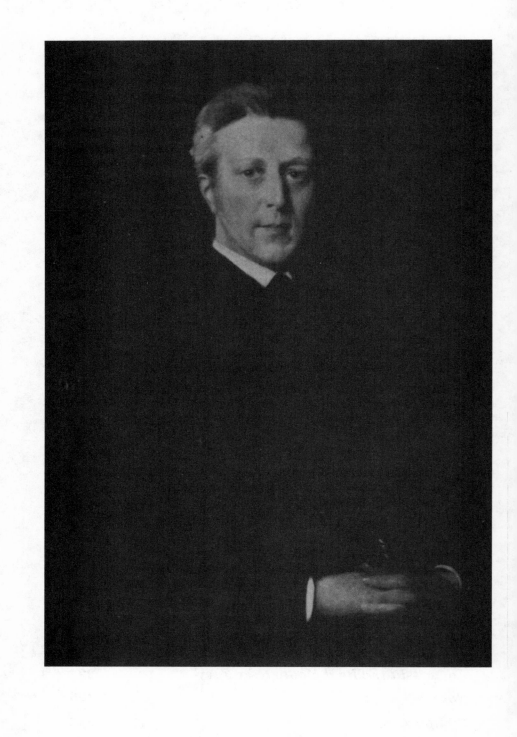

Introduction/Acknowledgements

That indefatigable Scotsman, James Boswell, set a standard back in 1791 for all future biographers. Few biographers were as fortunate as the young laird. He copied down Dr. Johnson's every word, noted his warts and eccentricities, gathered up old letters, and interviewed everyone who had ever seen the great Dr. Sam. His problem: what to delete. Few could be so fortunate.

Dr. Joseph Bell would have been appalled at a Boswell hanging on his every word. He was a man who valued his privacy. Though he kept a Journal there is scarce a mention of the luminaries who touched his life—Florence Nightingale, Joseph Lister, Ellen Terry, or Conan Doyle. He does tell his daughter about a visit from the Queen.

From the beginning I knew that he was not an easy soul for some contemporaries or a biographer to know, but when I saw what Modern Edinburghians thought of him, what his students and children said about him, a life of this noble man became a work of love—and great curiosity.

It matters little in this writer's opinion whether Dr. Joseph Bell was *the* model or *a* model for Sherlock Holmes. The Method he inculcated in his students and his family was fascinating, and was certainly the dazzling method that is the great detective's trademark.

What does emerge from the Journal is the picture of a respectable Victorian with a scalpel-sharp mind and amazing powers of observation; a devoted husband and father; and perhaps—above all—one who knew as surely as Edinburgh was heaven on earth that there was a more glorious Heaven to come. He was a church-going man.

I began the biography of this unassuming surgeon as an ardent Sherlockian. Today I find myself also a devoted Edinburghian; a medical history devotee; and one with an undying gratitude for some amazing people whom I've met mostly through the mail and generally from Edinburgh. They have not only told me about Victorian Edinburgh in their letters, they have shown me modern Edinburgh through their kindness, help, and encouragement. One, Miss Jean Adams, Reference Librarian at the University of Edinburgh, even told me all about a Chicago "gold mine"—the Archibald Church Memorial Medical Library, located in the heart of Chicago's Loop.

My wife and I were invited by Brig. J.N. Stisted and his wife Judith to be their guests at Sandhurst, England's early-day West Point. Those good people spread out Dr. Bell's Journals, his notebooks, his poetry on three huge tables, and turned their dining room, graced with portraits of Dr. Bell's ancestors, over to me. Brig. Stisted painstakingly answered my unending questions. They couldn't do enough for us. My debt to them is, like the towering statue of Queen Victoria at Sandhurst, monumental.

In writing to the editor of *The Scotsman*, Edinburgh's leading newspaper for well over 150 years, I met Mr. Eric Mackay and his secretary, Ms. Agnes Watt. They, with much encouragement, put me in touch with the BBC and helped me meet—in John Bunyan's words—two delectable mountains: Miss Esme Gunn, whose mother was a Dr. Bell-trained nurse; and Dr. James A. Ross, surgeon and sometime President of the Royal College of Surgeons, Edinburgh—a man who held many of the same titles and positions as Dr. Bell.

Miss Gunn has been a sheer delight. A senior citizen,

she has all the joy and wonder in God's green-and-golden world of a six-year old. She did more leg work for me in Edinburgh than Archie Goodwin ever did for Nero Wolfe. Dr. Ross, as I show within these pages, is a walking encyclopedia of the City of Edinburgh, the Edinburgh Royal Infirmary, and the Edinburgh medical scene.

Ms. Jean Guild, Librarian at the University of Edinburgh, has been my guide, my mainstay. Mr. Antony Shearman, Librarian at Edinburgh's Main Public Library, provided valuable information.

I cannot express my gratitude enough to Mr. Magnus Magnusson, whose charming history of the Edinburgh Academy, *The Clacken and the Slate,* provided me with nearly all of my information and knowledge about that institution. He has graciously allowed me to use material from the award-winning book. Mr. B.A. Stenhouse, Hon. Archivist of the Academy, provided me with records, information, and programs of the school. He was most gracious. Mr. Robin Price, Deputy Librarian of the Wellcome Institute for the History of Medicine, London, was also a cordial correspondent and source of information; as was the late Mrs. Eaves-Walton, Archivist of the venerable Royal Infirmary of Edinburgh.

Mr. Archibald H. Elder, of the Edinburgh law firm of Bell and Scott, Bruce and Kerr, W.S. (founded by Dr. Bell's brother), provided invaluable assistance. The Scottish Record Office and the National Register of Archives (Scotland) also were most helpful. I would also like to express my gratitude to Mr. J.T.D. Hall, Keeper of the Special Collections at the University of Edinburgh; and the Holmesian scholar, Mr. Richard Lancelyn Green, London. Mr. G. Dick, Secretary to the High Constables of Edinburgh, was most cordial and helpful.

In the village of Egerton, Kent, home of one of Dr. Bell's daughters, I tracked down Mr. George Pack whose father was a gardener to that daughter. Mr. Pack, himself a historian, was warm and hospitable, and had heard many stories about the famous white-haired doctor. He introduced me to Jane Sayer, who met the good doctor in Egerton when she was a little girl.

On this side of the Atlantic I have also had many kind friends and helpers. I was amazed and gratified at the generosity and assistance offered by four or five of the country's most knowledgeable Sherlockians. To John Bennett Shaw, who read *the* manuscript, offered suggestions, sent me articles, and encouraged me at every step, I am grateful. Others who went out of their way with furnishing suggestions, material, and advice were Peter Blau, Jon Lellenberg, and John Nieminski.

Mr. Irving Wallace, who wrote three early articles on Dr. Bell, not only encouraged me greatly, but also gave me access to many of his notes and papers at the University of Texas Library. I am deeply indebted to him. Ms. Ellen Dunlap, Research Librarian at the Humanities Research Center, University of Texas, provided much-needed assistance.

I would be remiss if I did not single out Sandra Choron, now an editor with Dell Publishers, who first suggested a life of Dr. Bell. I am grateful and indebted to Bernice Lee who waxed enthusiastic to Ms. Choron about me.

Closer to home, I am eternally beholden to Birdie Serlin, Secretary to Northeastern's English Department, who typed the manuscript; deciphered my crabbed longhand; made ingenious corrections; and did not blink an eye. She was magnificent. Kathy Snyder, also a vital part of Northeastern's vaunted English Department, helped out immeasurably. I must thank Dr. Earl John Clark, Chairman of Northeastern Illinois University's English Department, for his patience and understanding.

Northeastern Illinois Univeristy's reference library staff, under the aegis of Ms. Evangeline Mistaras, was efficiency and courtesy personified. All there were empathetic, eager, efficient. Sara Merens and Ann Wakefield make each day a joy. I would also like to thank Northeastern's Committee on Organized Research for a travel grant that helped get me to Britain.

The photography staff, especially Rich Sato and Roy Pope, proved of inestimable help. And, just east of Edens, I must pay homage to my driving friend and patient listener Irwin Glicken, who could probably assist today in any operation at any Infirmary.

On the subjects of publishing and the making of many books, I wish to thank my delightful editor at Popular Press, Pat Browne. Like many of the others mentioned above, I have known her only through the largess of the post office. It has been a pleasure to work with her.

Finally, as one who has been an intrepid reader of acknowledgements, I used to think they were like Mr. Holmes' 7% solution—helpful but not vital. Not so. For all the assistance of the people above, I thank them; for their knowledge, I salute them; for their friendship, I cherish them.

Ely M. Liebow
Northeastern Ill. Univ.
Chicago, Ill.
January, 1982

Foreword

It is a great privilege to have been asked by Professor Ely Liebow to write a foreword to his book on Dr. Joseph Bell. This task has been a true labour of love as my great grandfather has been a great favourite of mine since my earliest childhood. Although he died twenty years before I was born, I have felt always that I have known him. His almost life sized portrait, a photograph of which can be seen on page 171, used to hang between those of his parents above the sideboard in my grandparents' diningroom. Now it hangs on the stairs in our house in Edinburgh. I like to think that I can remember him from the age of three during my first visit to see my grandmother, his daughter, when my parents brought me back with them on leave from India.

To the family Dr. Bell was referred to as 'Gigs', a name by which he was known by those grandchildren who were old enough to have met him. To me his portrait displays a very kindly and intelligent individual, who looks down upon those who pass as a friend and confidant. Without a doubt there is a touch of sadness in his eyes, which seem to follow you as you pass on the stairs.

I have been brought up always to believe that he is the person upon whom Sir Arthur Conan Doyle based the character of Sherlock Holmes. My grandmother told me that she was convinced that he was the teacher who gave his pupil the original idea of that great fictional figure. This is borne out by one of the letters written by Sir Arthur Conan Doyle to my great grandfather on 4th May 1892, which is in my possession. In it he says: 'It is most certainly to you that I owe Sherlock Holmes, and though in the stories I have the advantage of being able to place him in all sorts of dramatic positions, I do not think that his analytical work is in the least an exaggeration of some effects, which I have seen you produce in the outpatient ward. Round the centre of deduction and influence and observation which I have heard you inculcate, I have tried to build up a man who pushed the thing as far as it would go—further occasionally—and I am so glad that the result has satisfied you, who are the critic with the most right to be severe.' I must not pursue this subject further as it is covered well in the pages which follow.

It is no easy task to sum up Dr. Joseph Bell in a few words. On the professional side he was an eminent and dedicated surgeon, who was held in high esteem by all those who came in contact with him. He was, without a doubt, a man of very high principles with a deep religious conviction. He was a strong family man, whose life was saddened by the early deaths of his wife, only son and eldest grandson. Despite these great setbacks he bore no grudge to the world and continued to do all that he could to alleviate the sufferings of others. He took a great interest in life in general, kept himself very fit by shooting and walking and loved the countryside. In his private diary, which lies before me as I write, he recorded the major events of his life over a period of thirty years after leaving school.

It has been a great pleasure for me to have been in a position to help Professor Ely Liebow in some of his research. To you who read on, be you Sherlockians or not, I can do no better than to commend to you all the results of his detailed study and research. It is a fascinating and human tale of a remarkable man.

Edinburgh   January 1982   J.N. Stisted

I

Afghanistan Perceived:
Being the Birth of a Model Detective

It was a raw November morning, 1878, and the lambent blue flames of the gas lamps cast a reassuring light.

"I really don't think you should keep the chap waiting. I believe he's at the door now and frightfully cold." The speaker, thin and wiry, was leaning back in his chair, finger tips pressed together, and his aquiline profile danced in shadow on the wall. Again he urged his medical friend and assistant to hurry. "Observe him closely, though, for he looked most singular dancing outside just now from one foot to the other."

His colleague, grunting and chuckling to himself, went to the door and admitted a bluff, husky man, with wind-chapped cheeks. The man fiddled with an old dusty cap and his face was etched with worry.

"You know my method," said the speaker. "Bring him over here to the front of the room and let us look at him."

"Good mornin', Sir," said the stranger, with a thick brogue.

"Good morning to you, my good man," said the wiry one, as his keen grey eyes took inventory of all his features. Again he turned to his assistant, moved a syringe from the edge of the table to a shelf, and said, "Well...what troubles this fellow, eh?"

"How in the world...sorry...I mean he looks worried, but they all seem to do that. His face looks chapped, but without a history or without hearing from him, what is there to see?"

"Ah, but you do see. Yes indeed you see, we all see, but often you do not observe." Then turning to the worried stranger: "Your back—it's your back. How it must ache, but carrying a heavy hod of bricks won't improve it."

The stranger, a hod carrier indeed, stepped back as if from a blow, and then asked in a quizzical, canny manner, "I'm not saying ye're wrang, but wha' tell't ye I was a bricklayer to trade?"

Sherlock Holmes interrogating a client? No. The scene was the clinical surgery ampitheatre at the Royal Infirmary of Edinburgh. The grey-eyed man with the "Look of Eagles" was Dr. Joseph Bell, an extra-legal instructor of clinical surgery. His uncanny diagnostic skills were so great that the students had never seen him make a mistake after that all-searching glance. In the third row, next to J.W. Beggs and A.L. Curor, Arthur Conan Doyle, entranced by yet another of Dr. Bell's uncanny performances, furiously took notes!

Without Sherlock Holmes few indeed would ever have heard of Joseph Bell; without Dr. Joseph Bell, there would be no Sherlock Holmes as we know him. Oh, what a thing is irony.

Arthur Conan Doyle, to stretch irony to its limits, wanted to be remembered as a serious writer—the author of *Micah Clarke* and *The White Company,* but if he had never penned the first Sherlock Holmes story, he might not be remembered today; if he had not seen "the face of my old mentor, Dr. Joseph Bell," as he tried his hand at his first detective story, he would have had a totally different detective.

Although Joe Bell, as he was affectionately known to his students and to all of Edinburgh, is inextricably associated with Conan Doyle, his life is nearly as well known to students of medical history and the history of nursing as is Doyle's to every detective fiction *aficionado.* And like Danny Kaye's movie that begins in the middle

for those who come in in the middle, we begin the private
life of this dedicated soul in the middle.

The year is 1886 and Dr. Arthur Conan Doyle is a
struggling young doctor in a modest home with a
prepossessing title: Bush Villa in Southsea. He had been
married less than a year, was making less than £300 a
year, and his first novel, *The Firm of Girdlestone*, was
being rejected by editor after editor.

Ever the Romantic and perennially the lover of
adventure, the young doctor turned to a form that he had
correctly analyzed in greater depth and detail than any
critic of the day, the detective story. Like his fellow
Scotsman, Boswell, Doyle was an inveterate journal-
keeper, and from the age of eight he let us know that he
was an insatiable reader, spending lunch money on the
works of Mayne Reid, Sir Walter Scott, Dickens and
Macaulay. Later he became fascinated with his
countryman Stevenson, with Edgar Allan Poe, Wilkie
Collins and the Frenchman Emile Gaboriau.

When he finally wrote his first line of detective fiction,
the image of Joe Bell at the university flashed upon his
inward mind, but Doyle forgot little and was not a waster.
In creating perhaps the most famous literary character of
all time he did not completely forget Dickens and Collins;
he owed much to Poe and Gaboriau; he even learned from
the French master-criminal-turned-detective, Vidocq; but
most of all he had learned directly from a deductive
master, a demon of diagnosis—Dr. Joseph Bell,
F.R.C.S.E., M.D. J.P. (Midlothian), D.L. (Edinburgh), etc.

In his autobiography, Sir Arthur himself tells of how
it all began.

I felt now that I was capable of something fresher and crisper and more
workmanlike. Gaboriau had rather attracted me by a neat dovetailing of
his plots, and Poe's masterful detective, M. Dupin, had from boyhood
been one of my heroes. But could I bring an addition of my own? I

thought of my old teacher Joe Bell, of his eagle face, of his curious ways, and his eerie trick of spotting details. If he were a detective he would surely reduce this fascinating but unorganized business to something nearer an exact science. I would try if I could get this effect. It was surely possible in real life, so why should I not make it plausible in fiction? It is all very well to say that a man is clever, but the reader wants to see examples of it—such examples as Bell gave us every day in the wards.[1]

For the latter-day pundits who would not take Sir Arthur at his word, and insisted that he himself was the model for Holmes, nothing in a sense could be further from the truth, for that view really overlooks the ingenuity that went into Conan Doyle's thinking. It was Dr. Bell who suggested Holmes' most dazzling and satisfying trademarks: the lightning deduction tossed off in apparent insouciance ("You've been to Afghanistan, I perceive," or "Beyond the obvious facts that he has at some time done manual labour, that he takes snuff, that he is a Freemason, that he has been in China, and that he has done a considerable amount of writing lately, I can deduce nothing else"). Doyle did not, however, forget the others.

He had spent his early years in vigorous exercise and vigorous reading. He had read not only Poe, Gaboriau, and Collins, but he digested them. Holmes tells Watson almost as soon as he informs him he is the world's only Consulting Detective, that "in my opinion Dupin was a very inferior fellow" and that "Lecoq," Gaboriau's detective, "was a miserable bungler." Doyle learned much from these two gentlemen, and resented remarks by those who could not separate his proud spokesman, Mr. Sherlock Holmes, from his creator. The esthetic problem, in fact, keeping the creator from his creation(s), bothered him so much that he penned an admirable poem on the subject:

Sure there are times when one cries with acidity
"Where are the limits of human stupidity?"

Here is a critic who says as a platitude
That I am guilty because "in gratitude
Sherlock, the sleuth-hound, with motives ulterior,
Sneers at Poe's Dupin as very 'inferior'."
Have you not learned, my esteemed commentator,
That the created is not the creator?

As the creator I've praised to satiety
Poe's Mosieur Dupin, his skill and variety,
And have admitted that in my detective work
I owe to my model a deal of selective work.
But is it not on the verge of inanity
To put down to me my creation's crude vanity?
He, the created, would scoff and would sneer,
Where I, the creator, would bow and revere.
So please grip this fact with your cerebral tentacle.
The doll and its maker are never identical.

From Poe's *Murders in the Rue Morgue* Doyle got his first-person storyteller. He saw the value of a faithful, silent companion-amanuensis. Poe's unnamed narrator was also no brighter than the average reader. On the other hand, Poe's M. Dupin was all forehead, all thought; he was eccentric; he read his companion's thoughts; he laughed at the bungling methods of the police. It is also likely that the retrieval of Irene Adler's picture in "A Scandal in Bohemia" owes much to Poe's celebrated "Purloined Letter."

Unfortunately Gaboriau is not nearly as well known or read as Poe, and Lecoq, far from being a "miserable bungler," is a rather attractive, ambitious young policeman, one of the Surete's finest. He is accidentally handed his Watson, his foil, a former cavalry officer with the delightful Gallic name of Father Absinthe. Like Watson, Father Absinthe undergoes a complete metamorphosis—from sceptic-bungler to faithful admirer, listening-post, protector.

At times Holmes' and Lecoq's language, actions and ruminations are so similar as to be frightening. We are hard pressed to remember which came first. Passages from Gaboriau's masterpiece *Monsieur Lecoq* have more of London's yellow fog that swirled past the ghostly gas lamps than the champagne-charged air of Paris:[2]

'What is it?' inquired Father Absinthe.   'What do you see?' 'Come and look for yourself, see there!' cried Lecoq.

The old man bent down, and his surprise was so great that he almost dropped the lantern. 'Oh!' said he in a stifled voice, 'a man's footprints!'

'Exactly. And this fellow wore the finest boots. See that imprint, how clear, how neat it is!'

Worthy Father Absinthe was scratching his ear furiously, his usual method of quickening his rather slow wits. 'But it seems to me,' he ventured to say at last, 'that this individual was not coming *from* this ill-fated hovel.'

'Of course not; the direction of the foot tells you that. No, he was going away, he was coming here.... He was standing on tiptoe with outstretched neck and listening ears, when, on reaching this spot, he heard some noise, fear seized him and he fled.'

The veteran would have given something if he could have found some objection to offer; but unfortunately he could find none. 'Upon my word!' he exclaimed, 'yours is a droll way of proceeding. You are only a conscript; I am a veteran in the service...but never have I seen—'

'Nonsense,' interrupted Lecoq, 'you will see much more. For example...study the man's footprints, and you, who are very sharp, will see at once that he deviated from a straight course. He was in such a doubt that he was obliged to search for the gate with his hand stretched out before him—and his fingers have left their imprint on the thin covering of snow that lies upon the upper railing of the fence.'

The dialog sounds like a replay of Holmes' first great explanation to Watson at No. 3 Lauriston Gardens in *A Study in Scarlet*. Consider Lecoq's next move. Everything is present but the deerstalker and the pipe.

Quick in his motions, and understanding how to maneuvre the lantern in according with his wishes, the young police agent explored the surroundings in a very short space of time. A bloodhound in pursuit of his prey would have been less alert, less discerning, less agile. He came and went, now turning, now pausing, now retreating, now hurrying on again without any apparent reason; he scrutinized, he questioned every surrounding object; the ground, the logs of wood, the blocks of stone, in a word, nothing escaped his glance. For a moment he would remain standing, then fall upon his knees, and at times lie flat upon his stomach with his face so near the ground that his breath must have melted the snow. He had drawn a tape-line from his pocket, and using it with a carpenter's dexterity, he measured, measured, and measured.

And all his movements were accompanied with the wild gestures of a madman, interspersed with oaths or short laughs, with exclamations or disappointment or delight. After a quarter of an hour of this strange exercise, he turned to Father Absinthe, placed the lantern on a stone, wiped his hands with his pocket-handkerchief, and said: 'Now I know everything!'

Following this, the young Frenchman, hoping to preserve the suspect's footprints, shouts to Father Absinthe:

'Make haste: get me a dish—a plate—anything...and bring me some water; gather together all the boards and old boxes you can find lying about.'

While his companion was obeying him, Lecoq armed himself with a fragment of one of the broken bottles, and began scraping away furiously at the plastered wall that separated the two rooms.

His mind disconcerted at first by the imminence of this unexpected catastrophe, a fall of rain, had now regained its equilibrium. He had reflected, he had thought of a way by which failure might possibly be averted—and he hoped for ultimate success. When he had accumulated some seven or eight handfuls of fine plaster dust, he mixed one-half with a little water so as to form a thin paste, leaving the rest untouched on the side of the plate.

'Now, papa,' said he, "come and hold the light for me.'

When in the garden, the young man sought for the deepest and most distinct of the footprints, knelt beside it, and began his experiment, trembling with anxiety. He first sprinkled upon the impression a fine coating of dry plaster, and then upon this coating, with infinite care, he poured his liquid solution drop by drop.

What luck! the experiment was successful! The plaster united in a homogeneous mass, forming a perfect model of the impression. Thus, after an hour's labor, Lecoq possessed half a dozen of these casts, which might, perhaps, be a little wanting in clearness of outline, but which were quite perfect enough to be used as evidence.

Later, hot on the trail of another suspect, Lecoq tells his awe-struck, elder companion, after Father Absinthe says the suspect will recognize Lecoq, "No, sir, he wouldn't, for I should disguise myself. A detective who can't equal the most skillful actor in the matter of make-up is no better than an ordinary policeman. I have only practised at it for a twelvemonth, but I can easily make myself look old or young, dark or light, or assume the manner of a man of the world, or of some frightful ruffian of the *barrieres*."

Finally, and not to belabor the comparison too much, M. Lecoq goes with Absinthe to get advice from Moriarty's opposite number, a retired Napoleon of Detectives, one M. Tabaret, called "Pere Tirauclair" or "Father Bring-to-Light" by the police themselves. The aging oracle advises him:

'You see, my boys, everything has degenerated in these days. The race of great criminals is dying out—those who've succeeded the old stock are like counterfeit coins. There's scarcely anything left outside a crowd of low offenders who are not worth the shoe leather expended in pursuing them. It is enough to disgust a detective, upon my word. No more trouble, emotion, anxiety, or excitement. When a crime is committed nowadays, the criminal is in jail the next morning, you've only to take the omnibus, and go to the culprit's house and arrest him. He's always found, the more the pity.... You are surprised because you know nothing of contemporary history. If you don't wish to remain all your life a common detective, like your friend Gevrol [substitute Lestrade] you must read, and make yourself familiar with all the leading events of the century.'

Doyle obviously absorbed much of M. Lecoq, but that eager young detective forms only a few of the sinews of the great detective himself. On the matter of disguise, for instance, we know that Sir Arthur was fascinated by the real-life adventures of that rogue-of-rogues, that criminal-turned-detective, that Gallic Jonathan Wild, Francois Eugene Vidocq. Actually Holmes' entrances and exits in disguise are far more reminiscent of Vidocq (1775-1857) than of Lecoq, and Doyle was undoubtedly aware that Vidocq was one of the models for M. Dupin.

John Dickson Carr, Adrian Conan Doyle, and anyone

else who suddenly declared that Doyle himself was
Sherlock Holmes (they were both pugilists; both fencers;
both straightforward, no-nonsense men; both smoked
pipes when "the game was afoot"; both solved cases that
were bungled by the official police force) certainly have
much explaining to do when it comes to the physical
Sherlock Holmes. That tall, keen, acquiline-nosed young
man in no way resembles the Watson-like Doyle. But
surely we may hope that the physical Holmes sprang full-
blown and full-grown from Doyle's mind alone. The eyes
and nose may have resembled Joe Bell's; the long, thin
fingers may have come from Vidocq's Memoirs; and
Browning even has a poem, "A Likeness," in which there
is a satin shoe used for a cigar-case in a bachelor's
apartment; but scholar after scholar and Holmesian after
Holmesian has carefully drawn our attention to Holmes'
similarity to Wilkie Collins' tall cadaverous, beaknosed,
hawk-eyed Sergeant Cuff, he who solved the riddle of *The
Moonstone*. Not to be overlooked is the scholarly
speculation that Doyle saw Holmes in the unflattering
rather unattractive image of Sergeant Cuff, and that it
was Holmes' best-known illustrator, Sidney Paget, who
gave us a moderately handsome, top-hatted Sherlock
Holmes.

When we learn that Doyle himself favored purple
dressing gowns; and probably owned a gasogene for
making soda (he favored whiskey and soda); was
melancholy; and enjoyed long, solitary walks, a timid
voice in the back of the brain may query, "Where-just
where—was the supposed genius, the inspiration of
Arthur Conan Doyle? Just what was original about Mr.
Holmes?" The answer lies in the mix—the curious,
blending of ingredients that came from Doyle's romantic,
adventuresome mind, but a mind withal that was more
open to innovation and science than the minds of most
Victorian writers. Worried by the dearth of patients, a

growing family, and the heady thoughts of a literary life, he heard again the crisp, authoritative rich-Scots voice of his former mentor Joe Bell: "From close observation and deduction, gentlemen, it is possible to make a diagnosis that will be correct in any and every case. However, you must not neglect to ratify your deductions, to substantiate your diagnoses, with the stethoscope and by all other recognized and every-day methods." Joe Bell gave Doyle the scientific method, the voice, the stoic face, but most of all the true touchstone, the aspect of Holmes that instantly and forever raised him above all other detectives and made him more recognizable than almost any other literary creation: the ingenious, insouciant, lightning deduction based on a thread, a wisp of smoke, a scratch that most mortals overlook, but to Bell and Holmes was everything.

"You have been to Afghanistan, I perceive," said the great detective upon first meeting Watson.

"How on earth did you know that?"

Holmes knew and Doyle knew because beyond them both was the Method of the Master Observer and diagnostician, Dr. Joseph Bell.

II

I Heir the Bells
or The Sign of the Four

The Bell family, a name that was synonymous with medicine and Edinburgh for nearly 150 years and over four generations, traced its lineage back to the middle ages, and while all the medical Bells were models of skill and sobriety, the earliest Bells are associated with moonlit border raids, swashbuckling males, and romantic legends.[3] In all probability Bells from Dumfriesshire came to Yorkshire in the train of Philip Le Bel, and thence they journeyed further north to Scotland. In 1292 Gilbert le Fiz Bel was deprived of land in Dumfriesshire probably by Edward I himself. Dr. Bell's ancestors were a fighting race, leaders of the Clan Bell in the old Border Times.

The family estates were designated Godsbrig and Blackethouse, both in the parish of Middlebie. One George Bell, a Covenanter and a rebel, was included in Charles II's Act of Indemnity in 1662, but was fined £1000 Scots, and this may have led to the sale of the family estate by his son Willie Bell. It was Willie Bell who was "the first that ever brak the hole and came in about the Kinmount," in the famous rescue of Kinmount Willie.

George's younger son Benjamin, who changed the Bell's Coat of Arms from three Churbells [motto: I heir the bell] to a sheaf of corn, was the probable model of Sir Walter Scott's Young Lochinvar. He eloped with Rebecca Graham, daughter of a Captain Graham and Miss Kirkpatrick of Closeburn. It was the Grahams' act of cutting the bridles and girths of the horses of the

Closeburn Clan that gave rise to the legend of the gallant young Lochinvar. Two other early well-known Bells were the unfortunate slayers of "Fair Helen of Kirkconnel," herself acclaimed as a kinswoman of the Bells, and it was an early Bell who was chief of the Clan and who had on his epitaph in the Graitney Kirkyard:

> Burnt the Lockwood, tower and hall,
> And dang the lady over the wall.

About 1750 a member of the family repurchased the farm home of Blackethouse, with its picturesque old tower, on the banks of the Kirtle, and also the adjacent lands of Cushathill. It was this Bell, Benjamin Bell, who was the grandfather of Dr. Benjamin Bell, the first of the great Edinburgh doctors of that name, a name and reputation that Dr. Joe Bell fully maintained.

Dr. Benjamin Bell (1749—1806) was a truly remarkable man, and one of those gifted physicians of Edinburgh who helped turn the city and the University of Edinburgh into the medical center of the world. He served as an apprentice to a surgeon in Dumfries, a Mr. Hill. He then came to Edinburgh to study medicine, and from that moment on the Bells became an Edinburgh institution. Within two years of his arrival, young Benjamin Bell was house surgeon in the Royal Infirmary, and was on the staff before he was 24 (a pattern Joe Bell would follow almost to the letter nearly a hundred years later). His success in practice was so great that when he died at the age of 57, in Newington House, today the Scottish National Institution for Blinded Sailors and Soldiers, he was proprietor, in addition to estates elsewhere, of most of those estates comprising the bulk of the area now known as Newington. Blacket Place and Middlebie Street commemorate this connection, for Blacket House was the home of the Bell Clan and Middlebie their parish.

He was the first doctor in Edinburgh, *perhaps the world*, to restrict his practice solely to surgery, a novel, daring act that was watched closely by the Edinburgh medical community. In 1782, only six years after coming up to Edinburgh from Dumfries, he published his *System of Surgery* in six volumes, a medical marvel that actually reached the unusual distinction of seven editions, and was translated into French and German. It soon became *the* surgical text at the University of Edinburgh, and was used widely by schools in England and on the Continent.

We have said he was a remarkable man. Early in his career, after a fall from a horse, he was laid up for almost two years. He took a farm at Liberton, just south of Edinburgh, and began studying the growth of wheat. He also began studying economics and corresponded with Pitt and Adam Smith on the subject; he also wrote a series of essays on the famous Corn Laws and cognate subjects which he published. He was offered, and declined, a baronetcy.

His youngest son, Joseph (1786-1848) entered the medical profession, and thus began the alternation of Benjamin and Joseph Bell as Edinburgh surgeons. Joseph's oldest son, Benjamin Bell, Joe Bell's father, was born in 1810, and seemed to gravitate naturally to medicine, specializing as a surgeon. He held many of the same positions his son would hold when he became a surgeon. In 1832 he became a licentiate of the Royal College of Surgeons, Edinburgh, and in the following year a member of the Royal College of Surgeons, England. In 1864 he was chosen president of the Edinburgh Royal College of Surgeons.

Early in his career he specialized in diseases of the eye, and devoted much of his time in giving his services to the Royal Dispensary and the Royal Blind Asylum. On December 14, 1869 the male and female workers presented him with a handsome gold watch "as a small token" the

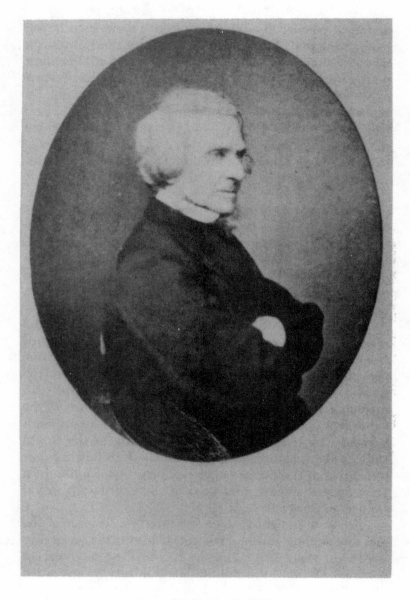

Dr. Benjamin Bell

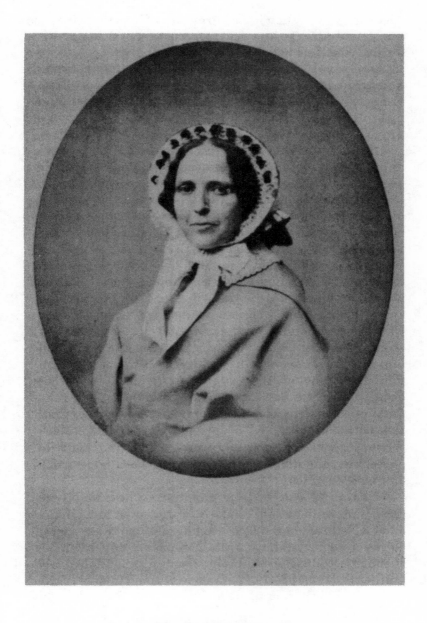

Mrs. Benjamin Bell

legend ran, "of their loving gratitude of his great kindness and attention to them for the long period of thirty years, during which he acted as their medical attendant, at no little personal inconvenience, and for a merely nominal honorarium." At his funeral in Edinburgh's Dean Cemetery "it was most touching to observe some blind men placing a wreath of flowers upon their benefactor's grave."

Joe Bell, man of science, lightning-fast diagnostician and analyst supreme, was a deeply religious man. The seeds for his fervent commitment undoubtedly were sown by his parents, especially his father. His father mulled over the matter of religion for a long while, but once he came to a decision, he never regretted it, stuck to the same path, and saw that his son got a deep, in-depth religious education. Religion in Scotland has always been an extremely serious, highly volatile subject. The good Scots not only fought with the English over the years against "the Papists," but objected to many practices of the Church of England, and even split violently among themselves over Church doctrine. In 1843 Benjamin Bell and his wife "went out" with the earnest Scottish ministers who "left the State Church not willingly, but because they 'feared God rather than man.'... They were zealous, consistent Christians," and the noble life of their first-born, Joseph, they "dedicated to God in his cradle." When Joseph came to marry in 1865 he and his wife agreed that a tenth part of their income was to be set aside "for God's service."[4]

He was the eldest of nine children, six boys and three girls, and while he said relatively little about them in his Journal (started in 1862), it is apparent that it was a close, deeply religious family with Joseph serving often as shepherd, counselor and physician to the flock: His brother Robert (1840-1912) was one of the founders of the prestigious Edinburgh law firm of Bell & Scott (today:

Bell & Scott, Bruce & Kerr, W.S., still doing business on Hill Street in Edinburgh).

According to the family history kept by his father we know little about him before the age of six except that while he was an infant "it was soon considered necessary to have a wet nurse for Joseph, and we were fortunate in getting a young widow from Dalhousie.... This was Mary Porteus who proved such a blessing to the family and never left us till her dying day, December 21, 1867." At the age of six he was ready for school. When Joe Bell would grow up, and follow in the medical footsteps of his three forefathers, the caduceus, the symbol of the medical profession, would become The Sign of the Four.

III

The Prior-y School: Not So Elementary

The roll-book is closed in the room
The clacken is gone with the slate,
We who were seventy-two
Are now only seven or eight.

Robert Louis Stevenson

The Scots took their religion, their whisky, and their education seriously—very seriously, and never more so than the glorious Golden Age of Edinburgh education—from 1830-1890. None went about it as a parent more seriously than Joseph's father. "Joseph went to school for the first time about October 2, 1843. We were tempted by the nearness of Mr. Macdonal's School... but probably it was a mistake.... He went afterwards for a short time, October 1, 1845 to the Circus Place School, and ultimately to Mr. Oliphant's School, where he became acquainted with James Candlish, John M. Bell, and Donald Crawford." These three schoolmates were soon to be three of the shining lights in Edinburgh's brand new prestigious Academy.

Something truly grand was "going up" when little Joseph and his classmates skipped along Princes Street to Mr. Oliphant's School. Work was begun on the spectacular monument honoring Sir Walter Scott. The boys played an Hibernian version of hide and seek in the foundation of the new monument, slowing down when tired of that to indulge in Nevie, a Scottish version of hiding an object in one hand, while all the gang sang out:

Nevie, nevie nick-nack
Which hand will ye tak?
Tak' the richt, tak' the wrang
I'll beguile ye if I can.

Edinburgh Academy opened its doors in 1824, embodying a curriculum that would be all but impossible for most college students today. Joe Bell and his classmates went from ages ten through seventeen. Later it was deemed advisable to give five or six-year olds special classes in Latin and the humanities.

The Edinburgh Academy deserves special notice not just because young Joe Bell went there or because Robert Louis Stevenson sang its praises, but because it was a unique institution. The brainchild of a small committee, it, like the King James Bible, was one of the few truly inspired monuments ever put together by a committee. There were probably several good reasons why a new prep or upper school was needed. The old high school, located on Lower Infirmary Street, had been founded in 1578 during the reign of James VI. Edinburgh had started growing far more rapidly during the Industrial Revolution, and the New Town citizens of Edinburgh of the early nineteenth century realized that for the sake of health and safety alone a new high school was needed. To the founders' and citizens' credit they also demanded a better education for their children.

While an Edinburgh High School graduate may have received just as good an education as his Eton or Harrow counterpart, he was not getting the true classical education of that English counterpart. He therefore would find it far more difficult to enter Oxford or Cambridge, and, as Sir Walter Scott, one of the champions for the new school, observed, his chances for a job in government, a job abroad, or even a good legal position were severely hampered.

The two prime movers for the Academy were two

liberal Tories—a political position that automatically put
two strikes and a sticky wicket on them and anyone of like
persuasion. The two: Henry (later Lord) Cockburn, the son
of a Baron of the Scottish Court of Exchequer; and
Leonard Horner, a linen merchant, knowledgeable
amateur geologist, and a pioneer in worker education.
These two gentlemen realized that with the onset of the
Industrial Revolution the world was changing. Labor
leaders were arriving from England by the trains full to
organize, educate and woo the Scottish labor market; her
natural resources would now be more in demand; and a
cultural renaissance had begun chipping at the shell of an
Edinburgh that was still medieval in many respects
despite all the canal-building schemes, new mills, water
projects and gas works. Edinburgh was not called Auld
Reekie for nothing. Dr. Johnson, of course, added to
Edinburgh's unsavory reputation. After Boswell lured
him there, he was disgusted with the nightly ritual of the
citizens along Edinburgh's High Street discharging the
contents of their chamber-pots, and at the same time
shouting what sounded like "Gardyloo" (or, "gardez
l'eau"). As he and Boswell sauntered through the misty
streets of Auld Reekie at night, the effluvia strong in their
nostrils, Dr. Johnson grumbed to his young Scots friend,
"I smell you in the dark."

Employment was still uncertain, "typhus was known
as the 'poor man's friend' because it regularly cut down
the number of hungry mouths to feed.... Smallpox was
endemic, although vaccination had been practised
successfully since 1801. Without public services of any
kind, with sanitation unheard of, no piped water, and
sewage chucked from windows into the streets, doctors
battled in vain against disease. General hospitals, run on
charity, were incapable of coping with the victims of
plague. Volunteer societies did their best: there were soup
kitchens, sickness and funeral societies, friendly societies

and dispensaries handing out medicine for the poor. But hospitals were just as ignorant of sanitation or hygiene as the populace. Joseph Lister with his antiseptic system would not be born until 1827. James Young Simpson was a twelve-year-old—and a quarter of a century away from the discovery of anesthetics—which was no consolation to those requiring amputations in 1823." Let it be said here that Joe Bell, who lectured to nurses, to young Arthur Conan Doyle and other young medical hopefuls on the need for cleanliness and antiseptic technique even before Lister's great work, would not be born for fourteen years.

In Oscar Wilde's words, however, one may lie in the gutter and look up at the stars. Literary, cultural Edinburgh was on the move. Journalism began to flourish. The liberal *Scotsman*, founded in 1817, began to compete with *The Edinburgh Evening Courant* and the *Caledonian Mercury*. The Tories responded by putting new blood in the sick *Scots Magazine* and calling it *Blackwood's Magazine*. In 1821 even a scandal sheet, the *Beacon*, a Tory journal, was started. It was so spectacularly slanderous, says Magnus Magnusson, "that its contributors were sometimes attacked in the streets; in 1822, indeed, one of its writers, Sir Alexander Boswell (the son of Dr. Johnson's biographer) was shot dead in a duel with a man he had defamed.... It was in this exciting and excitable cultural climate, in an Edinburgh where young Thomas Carlyle was taking private pupils and immersing himself in German literature, an Edinburgh in which, according to Sydney Smith, people even did their courting in terms of metaphysics."[5] It was in this climate that Horner, Cockburn, and other wild-eyed innovators, all lawyers—including Sir Walter Scott—proposed a new secondary standard of learning.

There was much opposition to a new high school, later the Academy. The good burghers of Edinburgh were not concerned that the proposed site at Canonmills Park was not overly convenient, or that access to it meant crossing many of the new busy thoroughfares; or that the boys might be in danger from the Water of Leith in times of flood; or that the school was sandwiched between Haigs Distillery and a tannery—no, the principal objection was that the new education at the Academy would put a halt to truly democratic, Scottish education on the secondary level in the Athens of the North! Charges were levelled, especially by Old Bailie Blackwood, the most vociferous opponent of the new school, that hereafter education at the Academy would take on a Patrician character.

One Alexander Peterkin, in a letter to the Provost wrote: "The projected scheme is calculated to separate, by a line of distinction very marked very mischievous, the higher (or rather the wealthy) from the humbler classes of the community." A more circuitous and earthy letter appeared in the *Scotsman* on April 16, 1823: "However manly and liberal may be the opinion of the many encouragers of the novel scheme, I am sufficiently uncharitable to suspect that it derives a very powerful support from the aristocratic feelings of many of the papas and mamas whose hearts sicken at the thought of Master Tommy being obliged to trudge through dirty streets jostled by all sort of low and crude people; triumphed over in school by the son of the shoemaker and beaten out of it by the son of the butcher, and associating with vulgar companions."

As Magnusson points out (and one can not help but feel it as he reads the history between the lines), even though the *Dux*, or leader of the class, in 1853 was the son of a master baker, the Academy from its birth reflected a class distinction, and "did represent the first major break with the democratic traditions of Scottish education." He notes, however, that Class was not an objectionable word in the 1820s, and discounting the truly poor who went to the 'Ragged Schools,' there was not much to choose "between the schooling of an advocate's son or a shoemaker's son when it came to coarseness and crudity. Cruelty, bullying and drunkenness were the order of the day at places like Winchester and Rugby, and the descriptions of the sanitary conditions at the new Edinburgh Academy, as well as the fights that took place during and after school, would give today's New Town papas and mamas a fit."[6]

The relatively new, revolutionary education certainly left an indelible mark on Joe Bell, and probably on most of the boys at the Academy, but despite the comment by his appreciative friend Mrs. Jessie Saxby that Joe Bell had nothing in common with Sherlock Holmes except his amazing deductive powers, Joe Bell did take part in most of the Academy's games—games that became as much a part of the Academy's great tradition as the educational process itself.

The big game at the Academy was a holdover from the old high school. It was called Hailes, took an amazing amount of space, and was a cross between shinty, lacrosse (of all things), and mobile mayhem. Each of the twelve players on a side had a clacken, which he bought from "Mrs. Jenny," the janitor's wife (the janitors year in, year out were each in turn called "Jenny.") A clacken was a long-handled wooden bat, with a flattened spoon-like end. As in lacrosse, the ball was to be placed on or scooped up in the stick and carried towards the opponent's goal. When the nimble, skillful player weaved his way past or through the enemy, and could hurl the soft rubber ball from the clacken up against the wall he scored a haile. He could get mauled or roughed up in the process, but in those early Academy days there was no other sport like it. Some idea of the rough-house quality of the game can be seen from Hailes rule 20: There shall be no hard hitting (Slogging). The referee shall decide when there is a slog, and a maul shall be formed where the ball [or player] was 'slogged.'

Players could charge other players at any time.

Years later one Andrew Beatson Bell in his *Reminiscences* said just what Joe Bell was to say when he (Joe Bell) took up tennis: "To my astonishment I found myself at once a tolerable tennis player, a fact which I attributed, rightly, I believe, to previous clacken practice in the Yards. With the clackens we learned to hit a small rubber ball with considerable accuracy, and the larger tennis racket and ball came comparatively easily."

Every boy carried his clacken with him to and from school, for it came in handy—as a weapon in playground battles and, as Magnusson points out, in "skirmishes with local boys (the 'keelies,' or 'cads,' as they were contemptuously called) on the way to and from school. It was also indispensable for trailing along iron railings, and other noisy pleasures."

Above all else, however, learning was to be the primary objective. Just a few years before, Boswell had bristled but admitted there was a touch of truth in Dr. Johnson's observation that "in learning, Scotland resembled a besieged city, where every man had a mouthful, but no man a bellyful." Sir Walter himself threw down the gauntlet on opening day. Not only would the lads become masters of Greek and Latin and of ancient history, but they would also master English (and Scottish) literature and criticism. This, he said, would avoid the error of creating "scholars who can express themselves better in Latin than in English."

It was a dignified, joyful opening day. Years later, Rector R.J. Mackenzie put the mood into verse:

Well nigh four hunder laddies thrangs
Upon the bonny opening day,
Moncrieffs, Bells, Balfours, Woods and Langs,
And Aytoun o' 'the mellow lay.[7]

And then he referred to Wise Sir Walter who introduced Sir Harry Moncrieff, the latter offering an eloquent and fervent prayer:

> And gude Sir Harry raised the prayer,
> And Wise Sir Walter made a speech;
> Frae Wales he brocht a man o' lair,
> The well-faured eident lads to teach.
> 'He'll schule your bairns,' quote Scott, 'for he,
> Has skelpt [whipped] my ain successfully.'

The man brought over from Wales to head up the Academy was the Reverend John Williams. He it was who was to schule [teach] the well-favored eident [diligent] lads.

The largest jewel in the crown of learning was still to be Latin, and during the first two years of the Academy's history it was the correct or true pronunciation of Latin that started many a debate, hundreds of arguments, and countless letters to the editor of the *Scotsman*. The Academy directors were well aware that the short-clipped vowel sounds that permeated the Latin speech of English school boys was not the real thing. The Scots with their broad A's, for instance, were much closer to the original. The young men themselves pointed out that their Latin was far better understood by their French, Dutch and German colleagues than was the Latin of their British counterparts. It was "curahtor" in Edinburgh, but "curaytor" at Eton. There was the case of "the pawky Scottish advocate John Clerk of Eldin, who was pleading the cause of 'curator bonis' in the House of Lords." When Clerk said *'curahtor bonis,'* the Lord Chancellor interrupted pompously: 'Curaytor, I suppose you mean, Mr. Clerk.' Whereupon, quick as a flash, Mr. Clerk retorted, 'I'm varra proud to be correctit in my quantities by such a splendid *oraytor*, such a brilliant *legislaytor*, and such a learned *senaytor*, as your Lordship,' dwelling long on the long *a* in each word." Sooth to say, the Directors agreed that it would be more practical for Scottish scholars to learn both pronunciations.

Young Joe Bell entered the Academy a few years after the much-praised new curriculum had had its shake-down cruise. What classes he had from age 10 to 17! His Latin ran from Virgil and Sallust in the fourth class to Juvenal and Grotius in the seventh; the seventh class mastered the *Nichomachean Ethics* of Aristotle and read from the *Book of Luke* in the original Greek.[8] "Nearly an hour every morning was devoted to Greek and Latin Composition under the eye of the Master," and Joe Bell's Master at the Academy was Mr. Harvey, assistant to the Rector, the celebrated Dr. John Hannah, who was installed in 1847.

In the Plan [or catalog] for the Edinburgh Academy of the year 1856, when Joseph Bell was in Mr. Harvey's seventh class, the following was stated for all to behold and digest: "The English, French, and German classes are placed under the sole charge of the Master of Modern Languages and Literature. The gentleman who holds this office has spent nearly the whole of his life in France, where he graduated in the University of Paris, and where he afterwards for some years held a Professorship of Modern Languages in two of the Royal Colleges successively. It is his duty, as to English... to lead on the higher classes to analyze the works of Milton, Shakespeare, and other classical authors and to the practice of English Composition."

French and German were started in the fourth class, and the young men read Voltaire, Racine and Schiller with ease in the seventh class. There were classes in Scripture Knowledge; ancient and modern geography and history; a thorough grounding in English literature (they read *Paradise Lost* and two plays of Shakespeare in the fifth class); natural philosophy, along with book-keeping, was started in the fifth class; and mathematics ran the gamut from addition, subtraction, and "vulgar fractions," to post-Euclidean geometry and Mensuration. Classes in Architectural and Engineering Drawing, fencing, and art were offered as extra-curricular courses.

Joseph Bell was a good all-round student, finishing fifth overall in Total Scholarship; taking first prize in Biblical Scholarship; a second in Greek History and Geography; and a second or third in Mathematics. In his Journal, his letters, and even in his poetry, Biblical allusions came as easily to him as his breathing. Asked to address the freshman medical students in 1871, he advised them to be patient with the results of science. "Be patient...and though the shield which you thought you had been armed with was powerless before the sword of Azrael, still your labours are not fruitless, your art not altogether a failure."

Most of the prizes were awarded on Public Exhibition Day at the end of the school term. When Joseph Bell sat down on July 26, 1854 on Public Exhibition Day the scene must have resembled a sort of Academic Olympics. The public was invited, and during the oral parts of the examination, professors, parents, educational savants, and sceptics could ask questions of the young men.

Most ingenious questions were thrown at the young scholars, questions that often overlapped several disciplines. An 1854 history question, for example, asked the young men to distinguish between *Rogatio—Lex—Plebiscitum—Senatus Consultam;* also they were asked to state briefly the provisions of the following, with dates of their introduction: *Lex Cornelia, Ogulnia, Terentilia,* and *Rogationes Liciniae.* In the Divinity examination they were to give the Greek words for *offenses—offend,* and suggest terms which would now convey the meaning more readily.

The citizens of Auld Reekie wanted their money's worth, but what is more important and more fascinating, they saw to it that they became involved in and stayed informed of the education of their sons. Their money's worth at the time that Joe Bell enrolled was the £3, 6s that was charged by the old high school, plus an extra guinea to be tacked on to defray costs for the new building(s). Ironically, the new "entrance fee" was also to be paid by the boys at the old high school. Both Magnusson and Lord Cockburn (in his Journal) break down the original costs:

4 quarters at 10/6	£2, 2s
Candlemas [gift]	20s 6d
The Rector	5s
The Janitor	5s
Coal Money	2s 6d
Library	1s
	£3 6s

Joe Bell said little of his days at the Academy. He did, however, dwell fondly on cricket and hailes; he noted the discipline; and could not help but mention two of the instructors who, though diverse as they could be, would stand out at any educational institution. From both of them young Joe Bell learned much, and much of what seeped into his very being came not solely from the classroom. Both were legends in their own day.

James Gloag, looking like a bulldog and full of chalk, taught math, and while more of his students went on to take more top honors in math (on a percentage basis) than the students of any other math master, his students remembered him for his broad Scots accent, his black suit with a tail-coat that was always covered with chalk; and his deadly accuracy with the tawse. The tawse was to the Academy what the whip was to Simon Legree and Captain Bligh; what the rod was to Jonathan Edwards; what the cane was to Eton. The tawse was "a leather strap cut into two or more thongs at one end. It was part of the canon of school dogma that tawses manufactured in Lochgelly, Fife, have always been the most efficacious."[9]

While the Academy felt the tawse should be reserved for extreme cases of disobedience or serious moral offenses, it was evident that "palmies," or strapping on the hand, were common, and that many masters, including James Gloag, were not averse to inflicting blows to other parts of the body. Just as Mr. Gloag's tongue twisted the language, so the boys were fond of chanting "Greasy Gloag loves to floag." The directors of the Academy never carried out their threat to dismiss him if he were caught once more and found guilty of striking a boy in anger. Once he admitted, when accused of belting a boy thirty times over the head and legs, that he may have hit the boy about ten times for not sticking out his hand.

As Magnusson tells us, he had a broad way with vowels, a way of speaking like no other soul. For 'road' he said 'rod'; 'rod' became 'road'; so "Get out of the road" became "T'oot o' the rod," and when he roared "Fatch the road," all the lads quaked in their seats at the "Fetch-the-rod" message. For inattention he always told the young offender to "copy doon the first sax sums on the board an' bring them nicely oot in the mornin'." (He always had a supply of punitive sums on the board.)

Long after the school abandoned individual class prayers for collective school prayers in the Hall, Mr. Gloag would start his first morning class off with prayers, "his piety, never quite proof against his devotion to math, for he would always finish the prayer with '...the Poo'er and the Glory, for ever and ever (tak up yir slates), Amen'." The greatest sin in his class, one that filled the bowels of his students with fear and trembling, was making a screeching noise on the slate with the ever-present slate-pencil. At the tiniest squeak of the skirl, Mr. Gloat would "bring down the road," but a long lingering skirl would have the Master lunging for his tawse in a fury. Since the worst sounds were made by the sharpest pencils, Mr. Gloag, a stickler for efficiency and perfection, saw to it that an old fashioned rubbing stone was used. It produced a softer point.

Magnusson brilliantly recounts the agonies of one of the new boys—Matthew Heddle by name—who produced a gleaming new pocket-knife one day and proceeded to sharpen his pencil therewith. He wound up with a stiletto-like point. He eagerly started working on his sums when—alas! The grandfather of all skirl-squeals came from his slate.

" 'What booie was that? Was't you? Was't you? Was't you? Haw, it was *you*, Haddle!' "

Young Heddle, perfectly unaware of any transgression (but beginning to tremble) held up his sharpened point and began to explain about the knife.

" 'Lat's see the knife, Haddle. That's a pretty knife, Haddle, a verra pretty knife!' "

Mr. Gloag then triumphantly held up the gleaming blades to the class; grabbed young Heddle by the collar, took him to the fireplace, and bade him take a last look at his proud possession—which he then dropped into the middle of the burning embers. But, as Magnusson recalls, the master didn't like the look of longing in the boy's face. "We've no' din yet. Fatch the tawse, Haddle." It may have been feared that the Academy was to be a School for Patricians, but for many of the boys it was a spiritual-physical-mental obstacle course. It was sink or swim.

The other instructor mentioned by young Dr. Joseph Bell was D'Arcy Wentworth Thompson, who was not Bell's master nor Rector of the Academy, but the Classics Master and a beautiful human being. It was D'Arcy Thompson who, following The Great Detective's advice, not only *looked* but truly observed. He saw lively, mischievous, frightened boys in front of him, and he was just the man for them, for he was in love with life and especially Boyhood.[10]

He had suffered much himself under the English system of instruction, and he wanted his boys to enjoy the classics. "Oh...those orders to write out three or even five hundred lines; a punishment as practical as the old prison crank, which was abandoned as being useless.... What senseless insult to a poet like Virgil, to make his beautiful lines an instrument of torture." D'Arcy Thompson was a teacher years ahead of his time. He felt the teacher should be a dignified, respected member of the community; a boy should be treated as a future adult; corporeal punishment was usually detrimental to the person at each end of the tawse, and did little to inculcate any true respect in the classroom. "Whenever I applied my lecture implement to a child's palm," wrote D'Arcy Thompson, "I was immediately conscious of a thrill, as of electricity, that ran from my finger-tips to the very centre of my nervous system; and sometimes, after the performance of such an ordinary act of duty, I would find myself standing before my pupils with a heightened colour upon my face, and a tingling in my ears; and to a looker-on I should have appeared as one ashamed of having done some questionable deed."

Magnusson, ever in love with the humane people and events at the Academy, recounts the story of a frail lad who was backward in his Latin and who was missing many classes on what seemed frivolous excuses. When D'Arcy Thompson grew stern with him one day, and told him that he looked quite well to him, the boy said quite earnestly, "I am really very weak, Sir; far weaker than I look." D'Arcy Thompson was touched by the tone of his words and the look in his face, and thereafter a strong bond of friendship and sympathy grew between them. Weeks later when another of the boy's absences grew longer than a week, Thompson was afraid to make inquiries. Then, one morning a solid black-edged envelope came to him. The young boy had died of a contagious fever, probably cholera, which was then rife in Edinburgh, and *the* dread disease. (It had already taken the life of the janitor, Adam Pinkerton, in 1854—a fact noted by Joe Bell and Magnusson.)

D'Arcy Thompson knew in his heart he had to visit the home of the thirteen-year old boy, but, having a child at home himself, he planned only to present his card—so fearful was everyone of the disease. The poor lad had lived and died in a boarding house, and the landlady begged him to come in and pay his last respects in person. Thinking of how dreary the lad's life may have been Thompson penned words that should have been required for all Educators and parents not only in Edinburgh but in the civilized world:

> I thought that the good woman of his lodging had perhaps been his only sympathizing friend at hand.... I felt thankful for the cord of sympathy that had united us, unseen, for a little while. But, in a strange and painful way, I stood rebuked before the calm and solemn and unrebuking face of the child on whom I had frowned for his being backward in his Latin.... So I determined...for the mild reproof that once clouded momently very gentle eyes; for the love I bore my own little one; and for the calm and unrebuking face I had seen that afternoon; that I would do as little as possible in the exercise of my stern duties to make of life a weariness to young children; and especially to such as should be backward in their Latin.

Those who did not succumb to Gloag's intimidation, the tawse, the gruelling academic curriculum, the fierce competition—academic and athletic—were, in Miss Jean Brodie's words, "la creme de la creme." Young Joseph Bell took the awards and medals bestowed upon him by the Academy and turned his thoughts to medicine.

IV

Edinburgh University
and the Royal Infirmary—
A Study in Scarlet

Like his great grandfather Benjamin, like young Oliver Goldsmith, and perhaps even like the mature Henry Fielding, Joseph Bell, having heard the praises sung of the University of Leyden in Holland, packed one small bag and decided to scrutinize the famous Dutch university. Unlike the others, he did not stay.

Since the University of Edinburgh school, its faculty, and its facilities were undoubtedly the talk of the medical world in 1854 and soon to become the greatest medical school on the Continent; and since Joseph Bell lived within a half hour's walk of the great university, one might well ask why the young man would consider any school on the Continent. As with so many decisions in his life, Joseph Bell went about everything in a quiet, deliberate, even scholarly way. He was already keenly observant, methodical and thorough. He deliberately asked for, examined and weighed the information he got from his father's medical colleagues about medical training in Paris and London. He was never sorry that he decided to go to the local university; he was eternally grateful that he spent the rest of his life in Edinburgh.

Joseph Bell became so associated with the University of Edinburgh and the Royal Infirmary and the University, especially the medical school, became so world-famous in Joseph Bell's time that part of its unique, bizarre history deserves repeating. It was a school like few others in a city that was unique.

While there were six faculties at Edinburgh—arts, divinity, law, medicine, music and science—none of the other five are slighted when it is said that the school of medicine gave Edinburgh a world-wide reputation. Douglas Guthrie, indeed, claims for it a place in the apostolic succession that passed from Hippocrates and his peripatetic school in Greece to the first formal school of medicine at Salerno, already famous during the Crusades. From Salerno, Dr. Guthrie (who it must be quickly and parenthetically said was himself a great medical and Sherlockian scholar) traces the history to Montpellier and Padua, whose celebrated students Paracelsus and Sir Thomas Browne immediately come to mind—together, perhaps, with the discovery of the Fallopian tubes, and then onward and upward to Leyden and Edinburgh. Edinburgh's first professor of medicine was Leyden-trained, in fact. Indeed the universally acclaimed Dr. Archibald Pitcairne, who left a jeroboam of claret to be drunk at the restoration of the Stuart monarchy in his will, taught at both schools.

The founding father—or earliest leader, at least, of the University of Edinburgh medical school—was the famous Alexander Monro, born in 1697, whose first course was attended by fifty-seven students. His son, Alexander Monro, Secundus, succeeded him in the chair of medicine in 1758, and occupied the chair for fifty years, during which time he lectured to over 40,000 students, the lecture being almost the sole method of instruction until Joe Bell's days at the Royal Infirmary. The Chair, which had already become the most prestigious medical Chair in Europe, passed to his son, Alexander Monro, Tertius, who proved to be something of a blot on the family escutcheon. Far less industrious than his two celebrated ancestors, he was content to use his grandfather's notes, and occasionally introduced a point with the naive recollection, "when I was a student in Leyden in 1719," although he was indeed not born until 1773 and had never set foot in Leyden.

Interestingly he was an adequate teacher and the first of a long line of Edinburgh eccentrics. Fortunately he was followed by better and (often) even more eccentric professors. First, there was Dr. Alexander Wood, better known as Lang Sandy Wood, a general practitioner who was often accompanied on his professional rounds by a tame raven and a sheep, and who was the talk of the day because he was the first man in Edinburgh to carry an umbrella. He was worried that the bird would get wet. Lang Sandy inherited the Chair of Medicine from the third Monro. Robert Knox, of whom we shall hear more later, was a colleague of the Messrs. Monro *secundus* and *tertius*, a celebrated extra-curricular instructor of anatomy and a man perhaps best known because he purchased cadavers from that notorious duo Burke and Hare.

Actually, the second Monro was the discoverer of the opening in the cerebral ventricles, forever after known as the Foramen of Monro. John Barclay, John Bell, and Knox were superb extra-curricular teachers of anatomy. Following Lang Sandy Wood in the Chair of Medicine was the aforementioned great grandfather of Joe Bell, the first Dr. Benjamin Bell. Following in rapid succession were William Cullen, the first man to teach chemistry and physiology in English (or Scottish) instead of Latin; James Gregory, one of the Academic Gregory's, a family that provided over half a dozen professors to Scottish education. It was Dr. Gregory's powder (magnesia, ginger and rhubarb) that brought fast relief to half the upset stomachs of the Empire. "As a lecturer," according to the *Quarterly Journal of Education*, "he was without a rival— dignified, eloquent, and forcible."

The sobriquets, encomiums, endorsements of the early professors were more than matched by the praise heaped upon some of the early teachers of surgery, especially allusions to their skill with the scalpel. Robert Knox, as a teacher of anatomy, may have been *"primus et incomparibilis,"* but John Lizars, who held the professorship of surgery in the College of Surgeons of Edinburgh, was "bold and fearless, almost reckless, as an operator." He was the first in Scotland to tie the inanimate artery in the treatment of an aneurysm and the first in Britain to perform an ovariotomy. Robert Liston, who vied with James Syme (Joe Bell's legendary mentor) for the Chair of Clinical Surgery, was the first man to perform an operation in England under ether anesthesia. He was "a tall man, powerful in form, dressed in a dark, bottle-green coat with velvet collar, double-breasted shawl vest [sic], grey trousers and Wellington boots" and one of the boldest and most dexterous operators of his day. Like Lizars and Joe Bell, he was lightning-fast at the operating table. "He could cut the bladder for stone in two or three minutes at most."

From the beginning, the University was keenly aware of the medical needs of its students and the sick of Scotland. The foresight, innovation, new courses and techniques were positively amazing. In 1791 Alexander Hamilton of Edinburgh requested the university senate to provide a General Lying-in Hospital. His pupils, unlike most other medical students in Europe at the time and anxious to increase their knowledge and experience, were allowed to help needy women and to give students practical opportunities to study midwifery and the newborn infant.

In the same year of 1792 Andrew Duncan, Senior, proposed the erection of a Public Lunatic Asylum. Completed in 1807, it became a model of its kind. Sir Alexander Morrison and John Conolly ranked with

Philippe Pinel and Jean Etienne Esquirol, both world famous in the history of psychiatry. Morrison was a pioneer lecturer on mental disease. Meanwhile Conolly may have been one of the least known medical geniuses of the century. He deplored the existing lunatic asylums, and made the point, little appreciated at the time, that the healthy mind had to be understood to cure the sick one. In 1839 he became resident physician at the Middlesex County Asylum at Hanwell, and soon medical men from the Continent came to see Conolly's newest innovation— the non-restraint system. "I do not hesitate to assert that the more insane [more seriously ill] persons would be cured if moral treatment were better understood and administered in time," he asserted, and urged that clinical teaching schools should be established at the various asylums.

In 1806 the curriculum of the medical school was further widened to include military surgery, and a chair of Military Surgery was established. John Thomson, the first to occupy the chair, and his successor, Sir George Ballingall, were both veterans of the French wars. Since Edinburgh was the only British institution that included such a course in its systemic medical curriculum, its graduates soon predominated in military medical departments and the medical schools that set up courses in Military Surgery. Meanwhile Thomson and Balingall, dedicated, enthusiastic teachers and with much experience, brought much credit and glory to the university. Thomson toured the medical schools in France, Italy, Austria, Saxony, Prussia, Hanover and Holland. In 1815 he was a staff-surgeon in Belgium and was at Waterloo. Ballingall, who had served his country as an army surgeon in India, Java and France, wrote a well-received book on hospital construction.

Before Joe Bell's birth five Edinburgh-trained doctors became connected with the Royal family (as was Joe Bell years later)—one was a physician to George VI; one was that king's oculist; one, Sir Charles Lucock, attended Queen Victoria at the births of all her children.

Edinburgh alumni made the most significant contributions to medical science. Richard Bright (of Bright's Disease fame), was to show that dropsy could be the result of kidney disease; Thomas Addison, pioneer of original research on appendicitis, gave his name to two diseases; Marshall Hall discovered the human reflex action; in 1809, Ephraim McDowell of Louisville, Kentucky performed the first successful operation to remove an ovarian tumor; and Philip Syng Physick was the first North American to wash out the stomach with a tube in a case of poisoning.

The first medical school in America was established in Philadelphia as a "department" of the brand new College of Pennsylvania, and fittingly enough above the entrance to the medical college was emblazoned the thistle, emblem of its debt to the country of its parent institution. It was founded by two Edinburgh graduates, William Shippen and John Morgan, to be joined shortly by two more Edinburgh alumni, Benjamin Rush and Adam Kuhn. The latter two gentlemen took off enough time from their clinical duties to sign the Declaration of Independence in 1776. America's second medical school, King's College in New York, was largely urged into existence by another Edinburghian, Samuel Bard, in 1765. Along with Dr. Rush, he became one of America's most distinguished physicians.

As if Dr. Joe Bell's direct line of ancesters wasn't enough in Scottish medical annals, one of the greatest medical geniuses of the nineteenth century was Charles Bell, a distant relative. He is celebrated among his colleagues and in medical history as a famous operating surgeon, not as a physiologist, anatomist, pathologist, surgeon and artist. Born in Edinburgh in 1773, he left his native city for London in 1804. In London he devised a working concept of the nervous system when all in the field was chaos. His theory and monographs still serve as the basis of all knowledge of the human nervous system. When sixty-two he felt he had to return to Edinburgh. "London," he wrote to his brother, "is a place to live in, not to die in." He had been offered the Chair of Systematic Surgery at Edinburgh and he gladly accepted. He was evidently a superb lecturer, an extremely gifted artist, and a delightful human being.

By 1825 Edinburgh was still light years ahead of England in surgery and many branches of medicine. Clinical medicine and surgery were, in fact, introduced into Britain at Edinburgh, and when Joseph started medical school they were still almost confined solely to the Scottish city. One Dr. John Haviland, in fact, studied at Edinburgh between 1807-09, and became professor at Cambridge in 1814 and Regius Professor of Physics there a few years later. He was the first professor of both subjects to give a regular course of lectures at Cambridge. In 1821 the Cambridge Senate made two terms of lectures from him a requirement for the degree.

It was, however, to the Dublin and London medical schools that Edinburgh's contribution was greatest. Thomas Beatty, John Cheyne, Abraham Calles, Dominic (later Sir Dominic) Corrigan, Robert Graves, James O'Bierne, and William Stokes all returned to Dublin from Edinburgh's ever-more-antiseptic halls of ivy. Beatty wrote much on and became an authority on medicine and midwifery; Cheyne became Professor of Medicine at Dublin College of Surgeons and was the founder of clinical teaching there; Calles became Professor of Anatomy, Physiology and Surgery at the same institution; Sir Dominic was physician to several Dublin hospitals and lectured on the practice of medicine. He was president of the Royal College of Physicians of Ireland five times; Graves became Professor of Physiology at Dublin; O'Bierne was principal surgeon to several Dublin hospitals; and Stokes was appointed Regius Professor of Physics at Dublin.

Suffice it to say that eight of the first professors of medicine at University College, London, had been educated at Edinburgh—among them several medical giants alluded to above, including Charles Bell, who founded the Middlesex Hospital School; John Conally; and Robert Liston.

Just before young Bell left Edinburgh Academy to enter the medical school that was across town it was already the most celebrated medical school in the world, with students coming from North America, Australia, the West and East Indies, Brazil, Portugal and even from Leyden. The frosting was added to the cake, as it were, by two revolutionary break-throughs just about the time that Joseph Bell was accepted as a student. Dr. James Young Simpson, beloved professor of midwifery and women's diseases, perfected the use of chloroform as an ideal anesthetic; and the great Joseph Lister, like Bell a protege of and later son-in-law to Dr. Syme, demonstrated his antiseptic technique to the world. In the years to come Sir J.Y. Simpson and Baron Joseph Lister were to be Joe Bell's teachers and colleagues.

V

"Gladly Wolde He Lerne and Gladly Teche"— In Pursuit of a Career; A Wife; A Hospital; a Brace of Birds

Arthur Conan Doyle was born twenty-two years after his celebrated medical mentor and went to the University of Edinburgh the same number of years (22) after Joe Bell. The university facilities, curriculum, and philosophy would change greatly during those years, but Doyle's own words and feelings about life as an Edinburgh student would apply to university life in the 1850s as well as the 1870s. There were boxing as well as billiard matches to be witnessed in rooms in Lothian Street, recalls a contemporary.[11]

The young men (we shall look at the few brave women students later) who enrolled at the great university at the foot of the Castle knew that the school meant business. There would be few frills, few creature comforts, no dormitories, and no social clubs as such. On the other hand, there would be long lectures, long and rigid examinations, and long assignments. The faculty was short on patience with the idle and the incompetent, and long on discipline. In the main, the faculty remained aloof from the student body, and there are many accounts of undergraduates doing away with themselves. One had to learn much self-discipline, Doyle noted, for once the timid young freshman turned over his £1 note to the bursar he was practically on his own. While there certainly was a number of required courses in the arts as well as in medical school, the students were free to attend what lectures they pleased (text books, especially in the medical school, were practically non-existent until the 1880s).

Conan Doyle credited the Edinburgh University, in fact, with instilling stiff doses of discipline in him. It was easy, he hinted, to carouse, to get by, to become lazy, but the young Edinburgh student by and large became, according to Sir Arthur, far more self-reliant and scholarly than his strictly English counterpart. "Our undergraduate society," wrote Sir Robert Falconer, another Edinburgh graduate, "was one in which 'men' (not boys) worked hard at intellectual pursuits."[12] He goes on to say that on his first day he gave the famous Professor Blackie, who taught Greek, "three greasy £1 notes to enroll in his class; the same to Professor Sellar of Latin fame. These two classes are all the tyro takes for the session." Aside from a few text books, the young man then buttoned up his purse. Eight or nine guineas would be spent at the most. It was still the custom then to pay the fee for each class to the instructor.

Joe Bell, of course, came from a fairly well-to-do family. He walked to school. Indeed, in an age well before jogging became fashionable, Joe Bell wrote of the salubrious effects of long walks. Ten-mile walks were as nothing to him, but in later years as editor of the *Edinburgh Medical Journal* he recalled the hardships of many fellow-students living in garrets, sharing basements, and filling nearby boarding houses. Bell, along with noted historian Alexander Grant, cites the testimony of University Principal Lee before the Education Committee of 1826. Extreme frugality on the part of students was the rule. Lee told of a third-year student who said his living expenses averaged about 6s 9d a week; this included room-rent and fire, which averaged 3s a week. He breakfasted on porridge and milk; three days a week he had broth and a little meat for dinner; on other days, bread and milk, sometimes potatoes and herrings. He had tea in the afternoon, but no supper. Lee knew one young medical student who never wore stockings, but merely gaiters. Anyone who has read R.L. Stevenson's descriptions of Edinburgh's winters (or who has experienced one) will wonder how survival was possible. Eric Robertson, himself a graduate, noted that among the University's faults "the students live in town as they lived at home, without the civilising influence arising from sociable concourse under the same room. No 'Commons' conduce [sic] to the amenities of their lives. Their food they bolt in silent solitary haste, as a rule, and society exists for them no more than on the hillside, except during an hour or two a week at the debating or musical society.... Their morals cannot be looked after. Even illness or death might come to them through hard work, and yet their teachers know it not."[13]

Many of the students that Joe Bell knew at the Academy came from well-to-do homes. At the University he met poverty face to face for the first time. His father, probably the doctor in Edinburgh who then devoted more time to charitable institutions and hospitals for the poor than anyone else, told his young son that he might feel proud of walking off with one of the Bursaries (or Scholarships), but that he would be depriving a needy lad of sustenance. Arthur Conan Doyle would wish in 1876 that all middle-class fathers would give their sons bound for medical school such advice. With his classical and scientific background there is little doubt but that Joe Bell could have a won a Bursary or two.

Like his celebrated pupil, Joe Bell had all the makings of a true Romantic from the time he could read, but also in the Bell household there were religious tracts and the Bible that he read as a young boy. He devoured the poetry and novels of Sir Walter Scott and from his earliest days

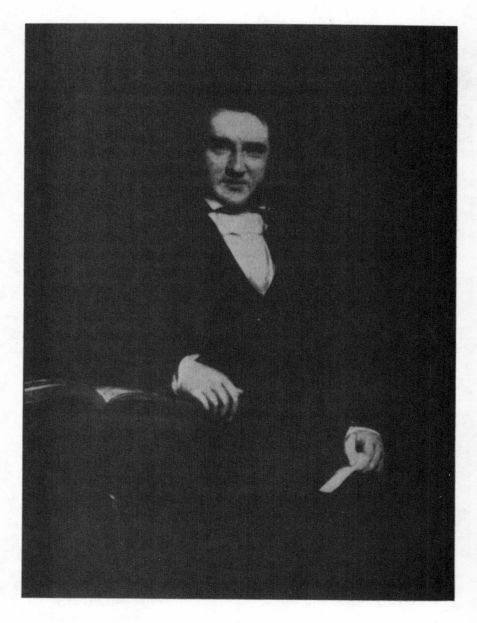

Sir J.Y. Simpson

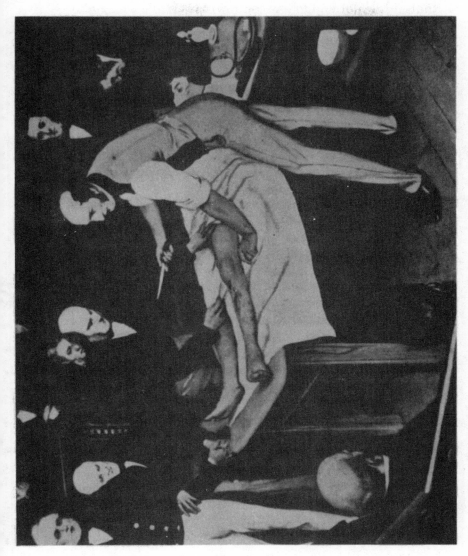

Robert Liston performing first operation under ether anesthesia in Britain, December, 1846.

at the Academy he began writing poetry reminiscent of
that of his idol and fellow-countryman. While waiting to
enter the University he started reading Browning, and
much of the poetry he was to write in later life seems like a
strange mixture of Browning, Scott and the Kirk.

If ever a young man was prepared to enter the medical
profession it was Joe Bell. He paid his "greasy £1 note" to
the Secretary at Edinburgh in 1854, and ran his eye over a
broadside announcing the Winter session, a session that
ran from October to April. On the Edinburgh faculty at
the time were, of course, many of the great names of
European medicine: Syme himself; Lister; Simpson; and
the great surgeons Spence and Miller.

Joe Bell, who was to devote a great part of the rest of
his life to the University, had little to say about his first
day or the next five years of medical school. The
University indeed must have seemed in part an extension
of the Academy. Conan Doyle, who lost the coveted
Grierson bursary of £40 on a technicality (the University
managed to find him "a solatium [sic] of £7"), began his
college days in "bitter disappointment." As he noted in
that sadly neglected first novel, *The Firm of Girdlestone,*
"The young aspirant pays his pound and finds himself a
student. After that he may do absolutely what he will."
Doyle recalls his college days rather ruefully in his
autobiography:

> Between [entrance and graduation]... lies one long weary grind at
> botany, chemistry, physiology, and a whole list of compulsory subjects,
> many of which have a very indirect bearing upon the art of curing....It
> was a strictly business arrangement by which you paid, for example,
> four guineas for Anatomy lectures and received the winter course in
> exchange, never seeing your professor save behind his desk and never
> under any circumstances exchanging a word with him.[14]

It would prove instructional and interesting here to
note that some inflation had set in from the time that
young Joseph Bell enrolled as a med school student and
the day that Arthur Conan Doyle paid his first four

guineas to his first professor. In 1854 the fees at the Royal Infirmary paid to a university professor or an extra-curricular professor (which will be discussed in detail later) was approximately £3. In 1879 the fees technically were for six months, £3, 3s; one year, £5, 5s; perpetual, £10 (a yearly price). Clinical medicine and clinical surgery each cost £4, 4s for the winter course, and £3, 3s for the summer. At the same time, the fees were slightly less at the school of Medicine, Edinburgh and the young candidates by 1879 had some choice.

A far greater difference between 1854 and 1876 was the prestige generated by the staff of the Medical school over the twenty-two years, and a phenomenal increase in enrollment. In 1859, Joseph Bell graduated along with 61 other medical students out of a total of 87 medical graduates. In 1881 approximately 575 young men graduated, and nearly half of them came from the Medical faculty. In 1859, approximatey 400 students were in the Faculty of Medicine; in 1888 (perhaps the height of Edinburgh's fame) the number stood at 1898.[15]

Later Doyle did admit liking some of the "remarkable men" who taught him: kindly Crum Brown, who taught chemistry; Wyville Thompson, the zoologist, and fresh from the *Challenger* expedition; Professor G.W. Balfour, "with the face and manner of John Knox"; and the most vivid, remarkable ones: the booming-voiced Professor Rutherford (the model of Professor Challenger); and Joe Bell. Bell too liked some of his instructors, but he stood more in awe (than Conan Doyle) of those he admired greatly—"the great Syme" and J.Y. Simpson; and he was somewhat more circumspect and reserved about the rest.

Doyle, who was trying to compress five years' study into four to save money, admits quite readily that he was "always one of the ruck, neither lingering nor gaining—a 60 per cent man at examinations." Joe Bell, who was more an 80-90% man, seemed to fret more about his immediate medical future. While still a student he decided to stay on at the University, and following the inclination of his heart and taking the good advice of one of his father's friends, he decided to stick to Syme. "When I was a first year student," he wrote, "one of the shrewdest of my father's friends said to me 'Stick to Syme,' and so I did, for five years."

It is relatively well known that Dr. Joe Bell chose young Conan Doyle to be his outpatient-clerk when that young man was his student. Bell too got his start in the same manner. Impressed with Joe Bell's natural curiosity, his keen interest in The Method (keen clinical and common-sense observation), the celebrated Dr. Syme chose Joe Bell to be his dresser at the Infirmary. Joe Bell and the Infirmary had already started a romance. It was to become a thirty-year inseparable love affair.

First, however, both young men had to take their final examinations. Doyle, whose 60% statement is attested to by many of his classmates, did a little better than usual, and Bell did particularly well in those subjects that had earlier given him most trouble—botany and chemistry. Years later Dr. Joseph Bell was to become an examiner to the Royal College of Surgeons, and he told his friend, admirer and biographer Mrs. Jessie Saxby that some of the saddest moments of his life came when the young medical students weren't making it: "I am now sitting in the President's chair of the College supposed to be watching the performances of a number of young doctors who are aspirants...and are writing answers to some very hard questions.... Some look unhappy, many won't get through I can see. Poor boys."

Conan Doyle, who may have kept more journals than his scribbling countryman Mr. Boswell, said little about his own Edinburgh finals, but he never forgot them. Sure enough, the protagonist of *Girdlestone*, the young, romantic, football-playing Tom Dimsdale, is a reluctant medical student at Edinburgh as the novel opens. For his final examination, he goes, in turn, before three dour, hard-faced examiners at three separate tables: zoology, botany and chemistry. It is torture to the young student, but vivid and effective writing. Young Dimsdale gives it his best, but the apprehension, the fear, the manner of the professors, and a final bucket of bones prove too much. Tom blurts out an inane phrase, and bolts the room to the accompaniment of wild laughter from the professors. Bell and Doyle, however, both gleefully put on a high crowned silk hat when they passed their first professional examination successfully—"To distinguish us," says fellow-student G.S. Stephenson, "from those who were left behind in the race, as well as from those who were just entering the fray."[16]

Young Joe Bell received his Medical degree in August of 1859. He was still but 21; more confident surely than many of his fellow-graduates, but also as frightened as many of the future. He had distinguished himself in his classics and surgical courses, and had developed a genuine love for Browning's poetry and a strong interest in the prose of Carlyle.

He had long been a favorite student of the great James Syme, the Napoleon of Surgery, and Syme was particularly taken with Bell's graduation thesis "On Epithelial Cancer," for which he received commendation by the faculty of medicine. Syme, the brilliant surgeon of whom Dr. John Brown of "Rab" fame wrote, "He never wasted a word, a drop of ink, or a drop of blood," took him on as his house surgeon and assistant at the Royal Edinburgh Infirmary, the great hospital attached to the University. At the same time the young graduate wrote "my cup runneth over" when he was appointed house physician to Dr. (afterwards Sir William) Gairdner. Acting on the precept strenuously enforced and encouraged by Dr. Syme that a thorough knowledge of anatomy was essential in surgery, Bell obtained from the celebrated Professor Goodsir the appointment of Demonstrator of Anatomy in the University, a position he held for two years. It was here at the very beginning of his career that his reputation for his special Method, his powers of observation, and his great teaching ability began to grow. Speaking of Bell's early days as demonstrator under Goodsir, Sir William Turner, one of the luminaries of the University in the nineteenth century, wrote: "Whilst discharging his duties he acted as my junior, and acquired a well-deserved popularity amongst the students from his powers of observation, his clearness of exposition, his capacity for taking trouble to help them in their difficulties, and by his words of encouragement."[17] Obviously some of the instructors at "Modern Athens," as Conan Doyle called the University, did talk to and encourage their students.

He put that "clearness of exposition" to good use in 1858. He was a member of the Royal Medical Society of Edinburgh, "the oldest students' Society in Great Britain and probably the world" at that time. Still not yet 21, Joe Bell read to the Society his dissertation on epithileal cancer, and was given a standing ovation, a most effusive gesture for a Society that could be most argumentative about business matters, but usually staid, stoic and hard to please when it came to lectures, new books, articles or monographs.

In 1859, not yet 22, he was the "president in the chair" of the Royal Medical Society. In 1860, while still house surgeon to Professor Syme, he wrote to Dr. J. Chrichton-Browne, the new president in the chair, "With the permission of the Society I shall have great pleasure in reading a monograph on 'A Case of Pulsating Tumour in the Orbit [the bony pyramid-shaped cavity of the skull that holds the eyeball]' at the first meeting of the Society after the Christmas recess." It was a monograph and a case for which the medical world was ready. He expanded his research on the topic later when his "Pulsating Tumour in Orbit Cured by Ligature of the Common Carotid" appeared in the *Edinburgh Medical Journal*, perhaps the most prestigious medical journal of the day. He was not too busy in October of this year to notice and applaud the opening of the first training school for nurses, the Nightingale School, in London. He was one doctor who from his first day on the wards realized the importance of good nursing, and the dearth of it, in the main, in Edinburgh.

The young man was far too well-trained at the Academy and University to be an all-work-no-play physician. Like Doyle, he tried his hand at literature about this time in his life, penning an article on housing styles for publication, and was delighted when *Cornhill Magazine* accepted it. While houses and gardens were to remain a life-long interest, he wrote no more such articles along these lines even though his friends encouraged him to do so.[18]

His own inclinations led him to delve into many other pursuits. At an early age he was greatly interested in all forms of nature; he was an ardent lover and grower of flowers while yet a young boy. Thin, wiry, with a shock of black hair, he continued his interest in hailes and remained an active cricketer among the Academics long after his student days. He began penning verses at the Academy, many of them on Biblical or Classical subjects, but a couple of themes were to run throughout his poems and letters the rest of his life: his joy in God's world; a Wordsworthian love of nature; and that pawky sense of Scottish humor that was his trademark most of his life. It was at this time—right after graduation—that he developed a deeper interest in world affairs: like Franklin and Boswell before him, world affairs was one thing in which, he told himself, he had to improve. At home at this time he began discussing medicine on a most serious level with his father (about to become President of the Royal College of Surgeons). He took to heart some words well-known to the Bell family, words that his great grandfather Benjamin Bell addressed to a young surgeon just starting practice in 1796: "Be not afraid of your ultimate success. I have never known an instance of anyone, in any profession, who did not succeed if he was sufficiently qualified, of industrious habits, and honourable in his conduct towards those who employed him."

If 1863 were not an *annus mirabilis* in the young graduate's life, then the fancy Latin term has little meaning. First, he decided to make his Journal a full-time thing, though in those pages as in so many aspects of his life, Joe Bell observed much, said little, wrote to the point, and established the fact that he was truly modest and selfless, and one who saw his strength and ability as God-given gifts.

He began the year with a Paean of praise to God and his wonders, for his family, his own fruitful work, and "E————, darling E————, lovely E————." It seems that at a party a year or so earlier, Joe Bell met Edith. While he (typically) said nothing about meeting her, he starts filling his Journal with "Took a long walk with darling E————; E————, lovely E———— and I, went twice to Church today; Darling E———— and I walked nearly to Granton." Edith Erskine Murray was a shy, lovely auburn-haired beauty. It is obvious the couple never doubted they were meant for each other. At the age of four, Edith suffered the loss of her father, the Hon. James Erskine Murray, son of Baron Alexander Murray, seventh Baron of Elibank. While trying to open up trade off the coast of Borneo in 1844, and while in command of the *Yonge Quene,* he let his guard down just once in his dealing with known cut-throat pirates and was killed. Thus, when the couple met, Edith was living with her mother, a sister, and a brother in Edinburgh on Ann Street. They announced their engagement in 1862, and two colleagues commented on the "absolutely seraphic picture" made by the two of them.

On January 11, 1863 Joe Bell joyfully recorded the news that "my Father was unanimously appointed by the University Court as assessor to the Examiners...at a salary of £100 a year." He little knew that it was to be yet again one of the esteemed positions of one of his forefathers that he was destined to fill in later life. The next day, "at a meeting of the Managers of the Eye Infirmary I was unanimously appointed Assistant Surgeon to my Father and Dr. Watson [sic!].[19] I trust it may be for my own professional good and eventually to the advantage of others." Four days later: "Today I passed my examination for the Fellowship of the Royal College of Surgeons." He notes that one of the professors made at least two mistakes in his questions. Bell, obviously aware of the slips on the part of the professor, certainly was going to forget the lapses, but the great Syme, also a master of observation, was watching Bell's reactions, and later, "Syme apologized for the professor." Syme, who predicted to all that Bell would someday become the Professor of Systematic Surgery at the University, advised him the next day not to read his thesis to the prestigious Edinburgh Medico Chirurgical Society, which Bell was invited to join in 1862, but instead to have it printed in the *Edinburgh Medical Journal*. Not a whit dismayed, he altered his plans by preparing his thesis for publication and gave a paper to the Medico-Chirurgical Society on the "Adaptation of the Eye to Distance and the Use of Atropia." Meanwhile, he was formally admitted to the Fellowship of the Royal College of Surgeons.

He would seem to be a young doctor on his way, but he was still a house surgeon, a position that brought no salary. He was seeing Edith as much as possible: "Today darling E————came to our house; we walked nearly five miles." He was a young man with a sparkling sense of humor, but undoubtedly thinking seriously of his impending marriage, his small salary, and which way to go. He went to Syme for advice. At the time, however, the young Mr. Bell could not have known that Syme was concerned about the career of his own son-in-law Joseph (later Baron) Lister. "He advised me," said Dr. Bell, "to stay at home another year to lecture on Surgery and then be guided by the amount of success and encouragement I should get whether to set up house in Edinburgh or to try a country practice, and also promised to do what he could to get me appointed assistant surgeon in the Infirmary for his ward." It is hard to imagine the young doctor ever thinking of practice outside Edinburgh, but he thought over Syme's advice.

Meanwhile Joe Bell returned to the classroom and Syme's wards, and it grew obvious that he brought something special to the classroom. He was not just another teacher. He challenged the mind; he was innovative; he insisted on observation, integrity and professionalism. He truly worked at teaching, and the students, used to rather uninspired instruction, responded enthusiastically. Near the end of the winter term, March 19, 1863, Bell records: "Today the students of my Tutorial presented me with a very handsome silver pocket case accompanied by a very kind letter," and then during the break, Syme advised young Bell not to press for an operative surgery course, but either Syme was cautious or not very quick in recognizing brilliance in the classroom. In any case, Dr. Bell was appointed to begin a series of lectures on operative surgery during the summer term. On June 22, Joseph Bell began what may have been the most inspired series of lectures on operative surgery in the history of western medicine—and literature.

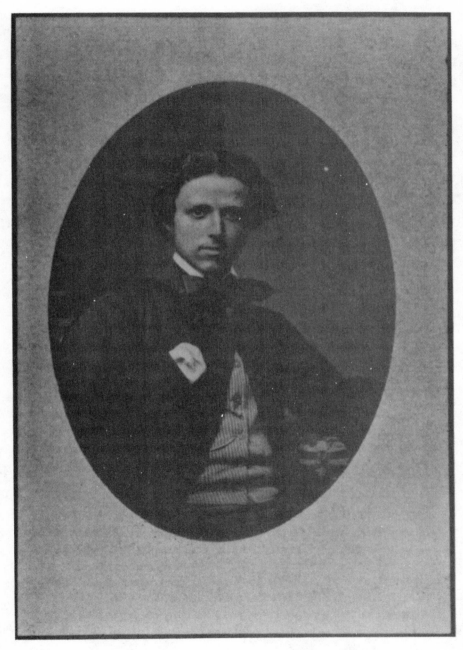

Young Joe Bell—with black hair. His hair turned white "overnight" when his wife died.

Life was becoming much busier and in some respects—more exciting. Feeling it his civic duty he became a "Joiner." In July he joined the Edinburgh City Artillery Volunteers, a Reserve or Militia formation. Dr. Bell's battery often took target practice with shot (grape shot) and shell (solid projectiles). On July 18 he shot forty rounds, and records: "We hit the target four times," but as an individual with a rifle in his hands, he had already become an excellent marksman. Ever since he was a teen-ager, he had been going to Glendoick House on the Glendoick estate on the southern slope of the Sidlaws, overlooking the River Tay. It belonged to the Craigie's (his mother's family), and was located in the midst of some of the best game country in the world—just east of Perth.

This was to be his greatest form of relaxation, and he diligently recorded nearly every one of his fall hunting expeditions. In September, 1862 he went to Glendoick and recorded in his Journal: "21 hares, 9 rabbits, 24 1/2 [sic] brace partridges, 3 brace pheasants and sundries—total head 90." He went shooting at Glendoick from 1863-70, skipping only 1864 when he was ill. In 1870 he started shooting at Glenogil and Pearse, just north of Dundee and about 55 miles from Edinburgh. He shot in the Glenogil area every fall from 1870-1889, skipping only 1875 and 1885. He started shooting at Corsock, just west of Dumfries, in 1875.

Like many a Scots hunter Joe Bell gloried in the profusion of game found throughout his beloved country. He was even more fond of telling the story about Ian MacDermott, a proud, 80-year-old who hunted every day of the season near the village of Pearse. Ian just knew that every game bird in the world was in the fields around him. One day an American professor came to Pearse and was astounded at all the spry oldtimers in the village. Going up to Ian as that worthy was about to go to the fields, he

asked, "Tell me, do you have many centenarians around
here?"

Ian, his pride and his mind racing at a furious pace,
pulled at his beard and said, "Well, now, I can nae be too
sure o' that, can I now-eh? We've always had lots o'em
hereabouts, but I did hear only yesterday at the Crown
and Thistle—our local pub y'know—that the very last one
was shot on Tuesday."

All the while the young doctor and his fiance were
making wedding plans. They had both been warmly
accepted by the other's family, and it would seem that the
doctor was from the first a favorite of Mrs. Erskine
Murray, and, as several of his colleagues noted, once the
naturally shy Edith warmed up to all the Bells they fell in
love with her graciousness and bearing.

In the winter of 1863 they took walks, long walks—
sometimes going over ten miles. They went ice-skating
together, and warmed up on hot tea, with perhaps just a
wee drop of something extra added. Above all, they went
to church together. At St. George's Free Church there were
always two services—one early, one late—on Sunday. Joe
Bell probably did not miss a Sunday service in his life and
often he would go twice of a Sunday. In the pulpit for much
of Bell's life was Dr. Robert Candlish, one of the giants of
the Church—any church—in the nineteenth century. He
was a spellbinder, a booming-voiced orator, and even
members of the Regular Church came to hear his sermons.
He was also the father of James Candlish, the *Dux*, or
leader, of several of the Academy classes that he and Joe
Bell attended together. In addition to attending St.
George's regularly and often twice on Sunday, Joe Bell
had much to say about the sermons, the hymns, the Bible
passages. "Nothing escaped him even in church," one of
his dressers said years later. " 'The Kerr child did more
than bruise his hip, but so far he doesn't know it.' He'd
often talk like that half to himself on Mondays."

That same winter Bell was sworn in as a High Constable. On his birthday, December 2, 1863, he noted: "Saw in the papers that I was appointed Surgeon to the High Constables." The High Constables were actually started by James VI as a kind of quasi police force to quell or discourage bully boys and vagabonds. Originally merchants or craftsmen, they later gave way to the "Trained Bands," a citizens' army of sorts. The trouble with both groups was that the good citizens could not devote much time to their peace-keeping chore. Over the years they became responsible for street cleaning, "an onerous task in a city that was, at least by repute, often as dirty as it was sometimes disorderly"; recorded the presence of strangers in the City; furnished annual lists of persons liable for jury service; and later prepared militia lists. In 1805 they became the High Constables, and "were called upon to act whenever Edinburgh threatened to lapse into the bad old ways of its riotous past."[20] He felt it his civic duty to join them.

Seemingly, with such a splendid background and start, one could not imagine that the young doctor, like Richard Cory, had his private doubts that none could see. He envisioned a "Chair" at the University; he loved teaching. He undoubtedly wanted to follow in Dr. Syme's footsteps. "Stick to Syme" now became "Be like Syme." The young doctor spoke eternally of Dr. Syme to Edith, to his parents, and even his students, and Syme was also on everyone else's mind in Edinburgh (as will appear below). Lister, Simpson, and some of the others are fairly well known today, but who was the celebrated surgeon, now nearly forgotten, who was a household word in Edinburgh and one of the titans of British medicine for over forty years? After Syme's death, wishing to commemorate a legend, the University archivist turned to the one doctor from the University who was known for his literary as well as his medical skill: Joe Bell.[21]

Bell's opening statement is as terse and frank as possible: "James Syme as an undergraduate did not take many University classes, nor did he spend much time within its walls." He got his Anatomy from Barclay, was a Demonstrator of Anatomy under the great Liston, but never took an MD degree. Not being able to "get wards," he courageously struck out on his own, starting a twenty-four-bed hospital, complete with nurses, dressers [assistants], and an out-patient department. He soon got wards in the Infirmary and the Chair of Clinical Surgery, "from which for the next thirty-six years [1833-1869] he taught Clinical Surgery as it had never been taught before, operating with daring, originality, and success."

Notice, as we bring Dr. Bell's account to a close, his economy of words. He combines beautifully the Biblical economy in relating a story with a classical arrangement.

The amputation at—or rather above—the ankle joint, which is known all over the world as 'Syme's' was an extraordinary improvement in the treatment of diseases of tarsal bones. Prior to his invention all such cases suffered amputation of the leg, deaths were frequent, and the resulting stumps were often fit only to be used with a pin wooden leg on which the knee rested. A 'Syme' well done is practically the only stump on which the patient can bear his full weight.... He was the first in Scotland to perform disarticulation of the hip joint. He perfected the methods of excision of the shoulder and elbow joints. He showed the way to the world in excision of the whole tongue for cancer. He was a pioneer in excisions of the upper and lower jaws for tumours.... Plastic operations on the face and eyelids he planned and executed with great success. He would remove a whole lower lip for epithelioma, and fill the gap by well-planned flaps, obtained from the skin of neck and chin.... He was neither specially dexterous nor specially rapid. In some operations, such as lithotomy and larger amputations, he was not at home from want of length of fingers and of muscular power. In all, however, his hands were absolutely steady and deft, the knife went exactly where he wanted it to go, and with neither haste nor hesitation:... And a little bleeding did not make him drop the knife and stop to tie the vessel, but he just went on, and tied them all when it was over. He had seen too much blood in the old blood-letting days, and knew that [little blood was lost] during an ordinary operation.... But all men who came under the spell of his marvelous personality will agree with the summing up of his qualities by

Dr. John Brown, who inscribed his "Locke and Sydenham" to his own master thus:[22]

'Verax
Capax, Perspicax
Sagax, Efficax
Tenax.'

[Veracity, Capacity, Perspicacity, Sagacity, Efficacy, and Tenacity.]

This was Bell's mentor, and just when the young man thought he was on his way to emulate 'The Chief,' he notes in his Journal for December of 1863: "I heard today that [Thomas] Annandale had changed his mind and intended to settle in Edinburgh after all, under Mr. Syme's wing—a rather black outlook for my future insofar as it depends on *his* help." This was just a week after dining with Syme, Lister and other colleagues, and feeling at peace with the world. Syme told a visitor about this time that both men would be future professors at the university. Joe Bell, reassured by his father and Dr. "Rab" Brown, decided clinical surgery and Edinburgh were the keys to his future success. He must work even harder.

On the first day of the new year, 1864, he suddenly found himself engaged in a peculiar undertaking— battling and campaigning at his father's side for a new site for the celebrated Royal Infirmary. Dubbed "The Battle of the Sites" by the journalists of the day, it would prove an undertaking that would—in one way or another—affect the work habits of Joe Bell for the rest of his life; the schooling and literature of Arthur Conan Doyle; and the healing of half the western world.

All things considered, Auld Reekie—or Edinburgh— may have been the most polluted city in Europe after the advent of the Industrial Revolution. A hospital in the midst of such a noxious place is going to have problems, especially since Lister's aseptic technique and Joe Bell's admonitions about "scrub-up" procedures were miles away. At the turn of the century (1800), "surgeons complained that during summer months the air was frequently rendered so impure in the vicinity of the fever-ward that the recovery of patients after operations was often retarded and that sometimes indeed it led to fatal results."[23]

New Town, as much of the rebuilding north of fabled Princes Street was called, was taking shape, and when in 1829 a new high school on Calton Hill was planned, the directors of the Infirmary, fearing the old school would be replaced by housing of skyscraper proportions, decided to buy up the old school. They rightfully wrung their hands, and said that unless the Infirmary bought up the Old High School, the circulation of fresh air could be cut off if tall buildings were erected next to the Infirmary. Thus they acquired the Old High School, as it was always called, and a site next to the High School for about £9000, and decided to convert it into a surgical hospital. Their first priority: an operating theatre that would cost an additional £3000. The new Surgical Hospital was opened in 1832. Some surgical patients, Dr. Logan Turner tells us, were still being operated on in the original Infirmary building, especially on Sunday mornings. Opposite the operating room on Infirmary Street was Lady Yester's Church, where the popular minister of the kirk and much interested in the welfare of his student-parishoners, deemed it wise to stop his service or sermon when the clang of the Infirmary bell resounded throughout the area, announcing the beginnning of an operation. The young men clattered out; the minister took his seat in the pulpit. "The lure of the operating theatre prevailed over the eloquence of the preacher."[24]

In 1833, following the purchase of the High School, the Infirmary took possession of Surgeon's Hall, built in 1697, when the College of Surgeons moved to their new quarters in Nicolson Street. They also acquired much of the property around the Hall, and slowly but surely were acquiring all of the legendary Surgeon's Square, birthplace and nursery of the extra-mural or extra-academical school of medicine.

The first lessee of the new Surgeon's Hall was Robert Knox, who succeeded the great professor Barclay as a professor of anatomy. Professor Knox, of course, is far better known as the man who purchased at least fifteen bodies from the notorious duo Burke and Hare. Since Joe Bell lectured (as Demonstrator of Anatomy under Goodsir) in the museum set up by Knox, and since Knox was, by all accounts, a fascinating spell-binder of a teacher, the young instructor, like most citizens of Edinburgh, knew all about the later career of the unfortunate anatomist. Knox was exonerated, but was in a kind of moral purgatory the rest of his life after the celebrated trial in 1828-29.[25]

In 1826, anatomical dissection had been instituted as a compulsary component of the medical curriculum, and Dr. Knox would need lots of cadavers for his many students. The transplanted Irishmen, William Burke and Willam Hare, came to his rescue. They by-passed the old body-snatching-in-the-graveyard trade by simply doing away with old, unwanted, unattached derelicts. "Fifteen times the devil's luck befriended them: the sixteenth turn of the wheel proved fatal to the murderers." The body of old Mrs. Docherty was recognized in Knox's dissecting room. Some said it was still warm. Burke was executed for the foul murders; Hare, having turned King's Evidence, fled the city. Knox tried hard to perform on a "business-as-usual" schedule in Surgeon's Hall, but the public's confidence in him had all but disappeared. What especially fascinated Joe Bell and his colleagues in the early 60s was the poetic justice at the end of the case. They all knew the final days of that infamous case almost by heart. When the gallows had been erected at the northwest corner of the County Buildings in the High

Street, hard by the old well, everyone wanted a vantage point. Even Sir Walter Scott got "part of a window" at the hanging. The poetic justice was Burke's dying in the same manner as his victims: strangling, suffocating, gagging. Irony was added when Burke's body became a scientific specimen after hanging before the public for over an hour. The body went then from the lock-up to Professor Monro's dissecting room the next morning. Present at Dr. Monro's lecture and demonstration (he was in his glory) on the murderer's brain was Liston the surgeon; George Coombe, the phrenologist (shades of Sherlock Holmes); and Sir William Hamilton, the philosopher. Professor Monro rambled on for over two hours, but so many medical students, not having yet seen the remains of the notorious Burke, rioted outside Dr. Monro's lecture hall. The police had to be called. Today a wallet made from Burke's skin is on exhibition at the Royal College of Surgeon's Museum.

After the trial, poor Knox became a lecturer in London, and then finished out his life as a showman to a touring troupe of Ojibway Indians, of all things. Echoing Chaucer, Joe Bell wrote a friend that he felt this was a case of the Fall of Princes. In addition to Knox's prominent place in Madame Tassaud's waxworks the lilting contemporary quatrain about the trio is what is best remembered:

> Up the close and down the stair
> But and ben wi' Burke and Hare.
> Burke's the butcher, Hare's the thief,
> Knox the boy that buys the beef.[26]

When the patients were moved from the old Infirmary building to the new wing in 1832, six surgeons were elected by the Managers to oversee the new Surgical Hospital. At this very time, the venerable James Russell resigned from the chair of clinical surgery, and in 1833

James Syme was appointed his successor. The Senatus (ruling body of the University) wanted him as a link, a continuum, between the Infirmary and the University. "As an old High School boy he was to become a 'Master' in the building in which he formerly sat as a pupil." Syme realized from the beginning that he was sitting on a septic powder keg. There was an abnormal number of fever cases in the wards, and the number of beds had to be greatly reduced because of the alarming rise in cases of septicemia and pyemia—both putrescent after-effects that were occurring because of the still-unsanitary conditions during and after far too many operations.

For years Syme, now one of the acting Surgeons to the Infirmary, fought for the construction of a new kitchen, laundry, and wash house, and finally a new, second surgical hospital. He began his campaign in the mid 40s.

In 1847, the celebrated surgeon Robert Liston died in London, and Syme was offered his chair of clinical surgery at University College. It was a great honor, but it was not easy for the great surgeon-teacher to leave a city where he was worshipped. He left for London in February, 1848, only to return to Edinburgh five months later. He felt they had not been honest with him about his duties and his work-load in London. In a letter dated July 6, 1848, Syme told the Managers of the Royal Infirmary: "If reinstated in the Royal Infirmary it will be my earnest and increasing endeavour to prove deserving of your confidence." Since the Managers were still in a state of partial shock from his departure, he was welcomed by the Managers and the entire Edinburgh medical community. Joe Bell remembers that his father drank a toast to Syme's return.

Syme returned to the attack as soon as he was back on the job, and in 1853 another new Surgical Hospital went up in April. Unfortunately, it was nearby the older Surgical Hospital, and since the number of incoming patients was on the increase, and since septicemia and pyemia were still on the rise, Syme kept looking over his shoulder as conditions got worse. In 1860, for whatever it was worth, young Joe Bell told his father the Infirmary should definitely move. When asked where, he gave an answer that would in the years to come prove typical of him—logical, cogent, and based upon common sense and keen observation: the Infirmary he felt should be close to the University and Surgeon's Hall; and the medical hospital and the surgical hospital should be centralized. His was his own, private opinion. Thinking the matter over, James Syme, perhaps in a display of pride, began expounding on the salubrious qualities surrounding his "old" Surgical Hospital. They had improved the air (by removing old buildings); increased the medical and surgical staffs; and were offering the best medical education anywhere. If, however, the present site were retained, then the houses facing the University should be removed, said Syme. Mr. David Bryce, considered an extremely competent architect, felt it would be a waste of time to renovate or build on the existing site. What to do!

In 1866 the best site for the Royal Infirmary was thoroughly explored and many witnesses examined. If the Infirmary were to remain in close proximity to the University, either the present site or the site of George Watson's Hospital—later called George Watson's College for Boys, had to be the choice. It should be noted here that George Watson's Hospital was situated on Heroit's Croft, an area lying between Lauriston Place and the Meadows, the latter an open expanse of ground.

While Joseph Bell very quietly was helping his father in encouraging the new site, Dr. Syme and many of his colleagues on the medical and surgical staffs of the Infirmary favored the existing site, praising the recent improvements. Syme, in fact, regarded the old surgical hospital as "probably the healthiest in Her Majesty's dominions." Objections were raised that the Lauriston Place site had many drawbacks, especially its distance from the University. Accordingly, in March 1867, a huge drive got underway to build on the existing site. In short order, over £110,000 was raised. A bill was introduced in Parliament enabling the Infirmary to acquire the ground and houses facing the University. Everything seemed ready for the groundbreaking.

In October, 1868, with ground-breaking ceremonies already planned, James Syme did the totally unexpected. He wrote a letter to the Board of Management. After recapitulating the course of events, he went on to say that "the sanguine expectations entertained from remedying the defects in the New Surgical Hospital, while certainly procuring considerable improvement, had not been realized, and pyemia—the scourge of unhealthy hospitals, was still distressingly frequent."[27] The language, a little on the Classic-jargon side, still made his point. Things weren't really all that salubrious in the Old Surgical Hospital. He went on to add that which Benjamin Bell had stressed from the beginning: while the new Infirmary was going up, Edinburgh would be without a major hospital for at least three years, depriving the sick of medical attention and the qualified of a medical education. "When the confined, smoky condition of the present site is contrasted with the airy, cheerful and salubrious site now within reach," he went on, "it is difficult to imagine what possible objection there can be to removal."[28]

A tremendous debate, of course, ensued, and Dr. Syme's most vocal critic was the celebrated Professsor of Surgery James Spence. Spence cited statistics that proved operations, on the whole, were most successfully carried out at the present site; Syme, just as vehemently, pointed out the relatively large number of pyemia and septicemia incidents, and the salubrious (it was a big word in the battle) conditions at the larger George Watson site. A vote was taken in March of 1869, and Syme's motion "for removal to the George Watson site" defeated Spence's amendment not to move by a 144-50 margin. Benjamin Bell was especially pleased, but rather appalled at the vehemence shown by the public and the press in the course of the debate.

It is highly probable that he may have been one of those who helped change the views of James Syme. Syme's *"volte face,"* as Logan Turner puts it, was a puzzle to nearly everyone. J.S., a Fellow of the Royal College of Surgeons of Edinburgh, recorded Syme's about-face a few years after the new buildings were completed in "educated Scots," as Joe Bell styled it, in the following lines of verse:

> So 'twas Hamish Syme spike it in a letter—
> If you want a site there is not a better;
> For ta air and licht are they not a treasure,
> An' ta price of all is just at your pleasure.

> Here ta patients wull, long perfore they leave us,
> Be as strong as kye [cows] on ta great Ben Nevis;
> For it's here they cure children's diseases
> Only by ta pure air an southlan' breezes.[20]

> Goot day to your, sir and what is it you've spoken?
> Had we not your word, Hamish, which you've broken?
> So you spurn ta place for your occupations.
> Where your great forbears did all their operations.[21]

Thus the young doctor worked assiduously for a new Infirmary, a hospital and school with which he would be associated most of his life. In the old and new hospitals he would perform countless operations; in the new hospital he would teach many young men, Conan Doyle among them, who would emulate his methods and, in one way or another, become his proteges. While he may have been most supportive of a new site, and worked hard with his father for it, he had his own life to lead, and in many ways the '60s for young Joe Bell were as tumultuous and earth-shaking as any decade of his life. By 1864 he was lecturing as an extra-curricular teacher in Surgeon Square.[31] On the wards, Dr. Syme was giving him more and more free rein. Almost from his first day on the wards it became apparent that the man with the look of eagles and the thick black hair was especially gifted in his treatment of women and children. They loved his gentle touch, his concern, his remembering all they had told him, but they respected his instructions. He always went over the patients' charts, and would want to know why any order was not carried out fully.

In the spring of 1864 Edinburgh was ravaged with as severe a diptheria epidemic as any city had ever seen. It was but the most recent in a series of catastrophes that hit the city. Writing in the *Scotsman* in February, 1960, the centenary of the founding of the Royal Hospital for Sick Children of Edinburgh, Professor R.W.B. Ellis noted that the "Water of Leith [source of Edinburgh's drinking water] was an open sewer in 1860, two cholera epidemics had recently occurred and a third was to follow. Louse-borne typhus and typhoid were common, and in 1862 there was an outbreak of smallpox. In the Tron area ["between the High Street and the Bridges"] the population density was 646 per acre compared with today's [1960] Edinburgh average of 13.9. Of every 1,000 infants born a century ago 146 died before their first birthday—the corresponding figure in 1960 being 25."[32] Joe Bell had worked overtime as a young assistant during two cholera epidemics. The diptheria epidemic was, he observed, even more devastating. He was working around the clock.

Joe Bell was frustrated at the gasping for breath of the children—the choking. They were, of course, being choked by the thick grey membrane at the back of the throat. No machines or instruments had as yet been invented to suction out the diseased material. The young assistant, however, developed a delicate, nearly flawless technique of sucking out "the diseased poisonous mass," by means of a specially developed pipette. Early in June, 1864, in applying his method—"late one night when I was amazingly weary, I believe," he himself contracted the dread disease. On Sunday, June 19, 1864, he records in his journal: "Since Monday have been confined to bed with diphtheric sore throat. Not much prostration, or anxiety but at times very considerable pain. Considering the dangerous nature of the disease (which I probably acquired by direct contact from sucking child Brittain's throat) I feel tonight wonderfully little wearied or altered for the worse since last Sunday." Then, in typical Joe Bell-fashion, he praises God and his parents. Syme, greatly alarmed, told him he needed complete bed rest. The young man was too sick to protest. Thus, he was sent off by his father to Glendoick.

In October, the first entry to appear in his Journal since July, he observed: "Last three months spent at Glendoick in a great measure as an invalid suffering from the paralytic sequlae of diptheria [a slight halt in his gait]—first in the throat and fauces [the constricted opening leading from the mouth and oral pharynx], rendering speech and swallowing difficult; next in the limbs, rendering me unable to walk or even rise from a chair without assistance and totally incapacitating me for some weeks from writing, from dressing myself without assistance and even from feeding myself.... I am nearly as well today [October 22, 1864] as ever I was excepting a little remaining stiffness in the legs."

A delightful piece of irony was played out in Joe Bell's own ward, "Dear Number XI," some sixteen years later when Queen Victoria came to visit Edinburgh. She spent two whole days at the University and Infirmary. She had heard many fine things about Dr. Bell, and was especially impressed with the rapport he had with the children. Dr. Watson, Patrick Heron Watson, told her the full story of Dr. Bell's ingenuity, his devotion, his bravery and his eventual illness during the diptheria epidemic of '64. The **Queen was so moved by the tale of his heroism that she** asked to have the ward renamed immediately. And it was. On the spot it was renamed "The Victoria." Felicity thy name is Irony.

Young Dr. Bell was, of course, correct about the virulence of his own attack, and the exact location. As Conan Doyle and countless other students noted years later, Joe Bell walked with "a curious jerky gait," and his high-pitched voice had a peculiar quality to it. Both physical changes were results of post-diptheric paralysis. Years later, in one of the clearest surgical manuals ever written for anyone (Joe Bell wrote it for his nurses), he commented on taking care of a child with diptheria:

> One word now on your duty to yourself. No nurse or doctor should think much of self or self-preservation. That is not our business, which is to cure our patients. Still no unnecessary risks should be run, and in tracheotomy for diphtheria [inserting a tube directly into the windpipe] it is right to remind you that both nurse and doctor run risks of infection, if by any chances the membrane or mucous be blown out of the tube [a newly devised one] with force, and thus enter either mouth or eyes. When the tube is being inserted there is generally a great rush of bloody mucous, so keep back your head; it is just the moment when you are apt to put it forward most eagerly. Also when cleaning or changing the tube, just keep your face out of the direct line of fire. Do not kiss the child at all, as your tender heart may wish to show your sympathy.

Dr. Joe Bell was not only a splendid teacher, but also very early in his career he was becoming the leading exponent in Edinburgh of preventive medicine, and playing a leading role in preventive medicine was the cultivation of one's power of observation; the development of one's common sense; and a new awareness of cleanliness.

When he came back to Edinburgh, he was still

worried about the future. On January 2, 1865 he "heard that Syme wanted to see me soon about a proposal which the managers were entertaining about appointing me as his clinical assistant surgeon in the Infirmary." A week later: "My professional prospects still look bad. Few patients, hardly any remunerative ones and class smaller than last year's." On January 23, much to his relief, the Managers appointed him as Syme's assistant. This position too was hardly remunerative, but the responsibility and prestige should certainly help with his own practice. He began seeing more of Edith; and to strengthen his weakened legs he set up his own training program of ice skating on Duddingstone Loch. Always an adroit athlete, he now took Edith on the ice, and their ten-milk walks turned into ten-mile glides, and gradually he pared the walking time from his parents' home at 8 Shandwick Place (they moved there in 1849) to the Infirmary down "to little more than half the time in a kind of canter." During this time of convalescence in the Land of Counterpane he too thought of "doing a book," a clear, useful manual for fledgling surgical students. He became excited by the idea. Also while recuperating he started following his own advice and became "more involved in world events." He became absorbed in the Civil War raging in America. The pages of the *Scotsman* were full of news of the war. Even though the young couple wanted to move the April wedding date up, Joe Bell told his colleague Dr. Chiene that he learned patience while recuperating. The day before he married, April 16, Joe Bell read President Abraham Lincoln's letter to Secretary of War, E.M. Stanton, dated April 3, 1865:

City Point, April 3, 3:30 p.m.

This morning Lieutenant-General Grant reports Petersburg evacuated and he is confident that Richmond also is. He is pushing forward to cut off, if possible, the retreating rebel Army.

Abe Lincoln

There were also three letters from Stanton and one from Grant himself.

The next day the Reverend Candlish, who rode with the young groom from Edinburgh, married Joseph Bell to **Edith Erskine Murray, daughter of the late Honorable** James Erskine Murray and Isabella Murray. Edith's mother, who had been a widow for over twenty years, had been invited by the young couple to live with them. Joe Bell not only respected Edith's mother, he was genuinely fond of her. It was his idea to have Edith's mother stay with them. After the untimely death of her husband in 1844, Edith's mother ·noved to 36 Ann Street in Edinburgh, only a few blocks from the Bell residence on George Street, and not much further from the third Edinburgh home of the Benjamin Bells at 8 Shandwick **Place. After a two-week honeymoon, the Joseph Bells** **moved into temporary accommodations at 1 Queensferry** **Street until their first home was made ready. On May 27,** **1865 the exuberant young couple moved into their first** **real home at 5 Castle Terrace, just south of Edinburgh's** **most famed landmark, the Castle itself. As with his own** **parents when they were wed, Joe Bell and his wife agreed** **that one-tenth of their income would be set aside for God's** **service. The young bridegroom had always lived at** **home—in Edinburgh.**

At this time Joe Bell became interested in two lines of pursuit (as opposed to hobbies) that would fascinate him the rest of his life: handwriting analysis and dialectology, the science of placing a person by his accent, speech pattern, or linguistic peculiarities. He was also becoming aware of the intense pleasure he was getting as a teacher, and in the summer of 1865 he "opened a new class of

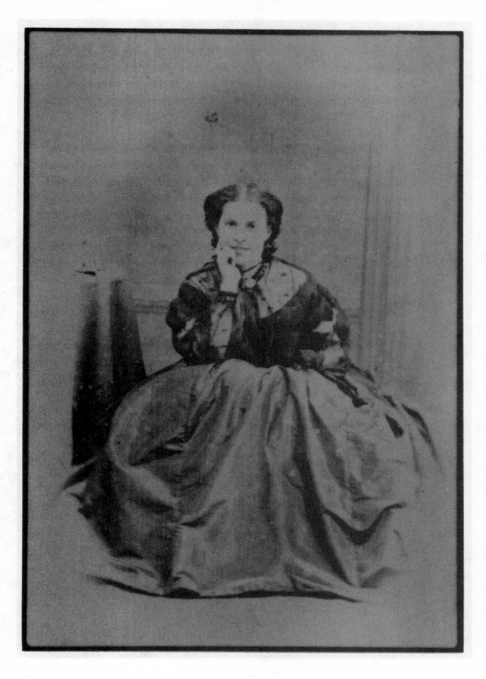

Edith (Mrs. Joseph Bell)

operative surgery." Thus, out of medical school for but six years he had already taught systematic surgery, and was now embarked on a course of teaching the more intricate and perhaps more involved operative surgery for the entire winter term.[33]

The marriage of Joe and Edith Bell seemed one that had been made in heaven, and if he weren't worried about the enrollment in his classes and the income from the private practice that he was trying to establish, the young couple would indeed have been living in an Hibernian Garden of Eden. In 1865 he records: "Only five students. Four more today. Laus Deo [a pet phrase of his]." At least three nights a week in "the wee library" he was working at "the little piece on surgery." He took enough time off from his writing chores to go out to the Glendoick Estate in September of 1865, and he recorded 24 hares, 6 rabbits, 26 1/2 partridges, 4 pheasants, and 2 sundries. In all his years of recording his catch he never expounded on the "sundries." On January 18, 1866 "a little lassie was born." This was Jean, the first of three children. The couple was ecstatic. On Sunday, January 21, they went to both services at St. George's (long a custom of Benjamin Bell and family) and they "cooked no meal that day." In the mid and late nineteenth century, there were usually two services every Sunday in most of the Free Churches—a morning and evening service, and usually a cold meal was eaten in between. "In the stricter congregations," according to Dr. James Ross, Sometime President of the Royal College of Surgeons, Edinburgh, and a veritable fount of medical and historical knowledge, "no cooking was allowed, a contrast to the modern 'Sunday Joint'."

On July 27, 1866, in his typically stoic style, Joe Bell recorded in his diary: "My book came out." This was his *Manual of Operations of Surgery for the Use of Senior Students and Junior Practitioners*. Published by

Maclachlan and Stewart, one of Edinburgh's three largest publishing companies, the book was well reviewed and, even more important, seemed to fill a real need of the advanced surgical student. The second edition of the book was reviewed in *The Edinburgh Medical Journal* of January, 1869. The tone and critical appraisal of the review would be repeated over the years for many new editions of Dr. Bell's books:

> In the present rage for writing big books on small subjects, thoroughly exhausting what might, could, would, or should be said in connexion with the text, but also the patience of the reader, it is refreshing to take up Dr. Joseph Bell's little work [267 pages], written in a condensed and vigorous style, and to wonder how he has managed to bring into so small a compass so large an amount of well-selected, practical information.
>
> As a guide for students or a memorandum for junior practitioners, Dr. Bell's book contains just the kind and amount of information which is required.
>
> The fact of a second edition being so soon called for, proves that its excellence as a Manual of Operations in Surgery has been fully appreciated.

Another aspect of the book that has been little appreciated is the similarity in style and tone in Dr. Bell's numerous citations of well-known and not so well-known operations with Sherlock Holmes' ticking off the great criminal capers of the past:

> It was not till the publication of Mr. Syme's monograph on the excision of diseased hip joints, in 1831, that the importance and value of the discovery were fairly brought before the profession; and the conservative surgery, of which excision as preferred to amputation is the great type, must ever be associated with British surgeons—Syme, Fergusson, Mackenzie, Jones of Jersey, Butcher of Dublin.

Jones of Jersey and Butcher of Dublin. Real Baker Street names. Indeed, some of the famous early surgeons, including one Timothy Holmes, author of the three-volume *Holmes's System of Surgery,* may have kept the undertakers as busy as the names on Sherlock Holmes' list:

> Mr. Holmes's statistics are interesting. He has operated on no fewer than nineteen cases [excision of the hip-joint]. Of these seven died, one after secondary amputation of the hip. Another required amputation and recovered. Two others died of other diseases without having used their limb. Of the remaining nine, three were perfectly successful, four were promising cases, and two unpromising [sounds more like the old Chicago White Sox].... Professor Spence in 19 cases had six deaths, or a mortality of 31.6 per cent. Culbertson's collection gives out of 426 cases, 192 deaths, or 45 per cent.

Above all, Joe Bell knew that a clear, concise manual on surgery would be welcomed by and useful to students. The success of the first edition and the favorable reviews did much to lift his spirits. Dr. Syme was especially pleased at the reception of the book. The young author knew the book could only help his professional career at the Infirmary. With a spirit far more blithe, and with his little black bag stuffed with letters relating to the handwriting analysis, he took the train to Glendoick in early September of '67 and recorded 20 hares, 19 1/2 brace partridges, 41 rabbits, 2 woodchuck. In his Journal he said that he was genuinely grateful for the past year, and eagerly looking forward to the new year. On the 12th of January "a little girl was born." Their second daughter was named Cecilia, but always called Cecil. "I am very thankful," he wrote. Two days later he was elected Deputy Superintendent of the Special Constables. Also starting at this time he began attending far more battalion drills. "Today Battalion Drill. Blank firing." He also became even more of a joiner by this time, serving as one of the founders, along with several well-known Edinburgh physicians, of the Round-Table Club, and served as its first secretary. It was a medical society devoted to good fellowship, good food and good medical talk. Papers were delivered, books reviewed, and often the give-and-take was heated. The summer class that year began on May 4. He noted that he had twelve students. "Be thankful," he said. A few days later six more students signed up. "Laus Deo."

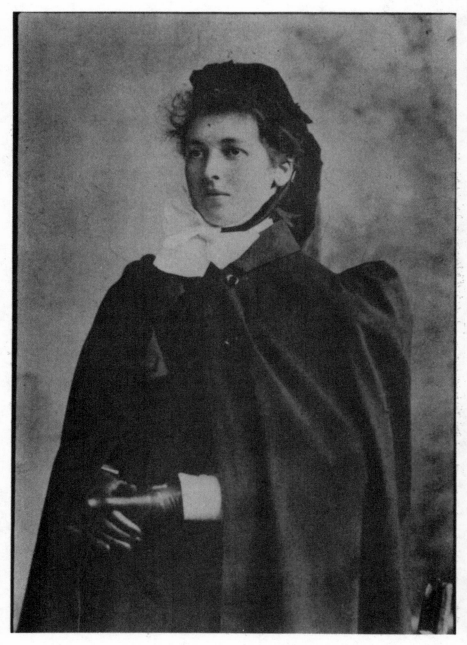

Miss Isabelle Jamieson, nurse trained by Joe Bell. Photo courtesy Miss Esme Gunn.

VI

Here's to the Women: Queen Victoria, Florence Nightingale, Sophia Jex-Blake, the Nurses, the Medical Hopefuls

One day during the middle of the 1868 summer term young Dr. Bell got permission to begin holding classes for the nurses at the Infirmary. It was his idea. He knew that many of the nurses were looking "for a warm place in winter"; many in 1868 had nowhere else to turn; they had almost no training; the patients suffered from their lack of training. Someone should do something. Almost unannounced, and at approximately the same time that Florence Nightingale was beginning her great nurses' training program at St. Thomas' Hospital in London, Joe Bell became a one-man school for nurses in Edinburgh. For once in the life of this notoriously private individual there is much to be found on a subject concerning him because every account of the history of nursing in Scotland at this time was turned over to Joe Bell. In 1892, at the insistent urging of the entire Scottish Medical profession, he turned out his succinct monograph, *The Surgical Side of the Royal Infirmary, 1854-1892.* Half of it was the history of nursing in Edinburgh. When Joe Bell came onto the wards of the Infirmary, the nursing profession as we know it was non-existent. Ever since the destruction and suppression of monasteries, there was practically no professional or skilled nursing in England—no one to take the place of the Mother Superior and the nuns who made up the nursing staff in medieval times (it is interesting, however, said Joe Bell, that the terms Matron and Sister never completely died out). The status of the nurse sank to an all-time low-level during the eighteenth and nineteenth centuries.

At the start of the nineteenth century many of the nurses were regarded as servants and attendants. They were poorly housed, poorly fed, poorly trained (often untrained), and they had gotten an evil reputation based mainly on the kinds of women who entered the field at the start of the century. In 1800 the nurses' annual salary rose from £3, 10s to £5 a year, while night nurses, who slept outside the hospital and paid rent for their quarters, saw their salaries raised from fourpence to sixpence a night. Joe Bell's account of things from 1859 on does not make for joyous reading, but as ever he was forthright, terse, perceptive.

A staff of nine women took charge of Dr. Symes' seventy-two patients on six wards and six tiny rooms. The two staff nurses were each responsible for thirty-six beds. And there were, says Joe Bell, "seven so-called night nurses who also had to do the scrubbing and cleaning of the wards and passages. The two nurses, Mrs. Lambert and Mrs. Porter, were wonderful women, of great natural ability and strong Scotch sense and capacity, of immense experience, and great kindliness." Then, like everyone else who breathed the name of Mrs. Sara Porter, who served under Syme, Lister and Annandale at the Infirmary for over forty-seven years, he quotes Henley's immortal lines about her:[31]

Staff Nurse: Old Style

The great masters of the commonplace,
Rembrandt and good Sir Walter—only these
Could paint her all to you; experienced ease,
And antique liveliness, and ponderous grace;

The sweet old roses of her sunken face;
The depth and malice of her sly grey eyes;
The broad Scots tongue that flatters, scolds, defies;
The thick Scots wit that fells you like a mace.

Much is she worth, and even more is made of her,
Patients and students hold her very dear.

But the other seven—"poor old useless drudges, half-charwoman, half field-worker, rarely keeping their places for any length of time, absolutely ignorant, almost invariably drunken, sometimes deaf...these had to take charge of our operation cases when the staff nurses went off duty." So wrote Joe Bell as historian. At the time he knew a radical change would have to be effected, for when he concludes his account, one can hear the anguish, the concern of a compassionate, devoted surgeon:

Poor creatures, they had a hard life. Their day's work began at eleven p.m., when in a mournful procession, each with a blanket round her shoulders, walked to their wards from a dormitory, so-called....They were on duty until five p.m. the next evening. They had to cook and serve breakfast, make the fire, help at the meals of dinner and tea. What wonder that at night they snored by the fire.... Serious operations were doubled in risk by want of ordinary care; haemorrhages were unnoticed, amputation cases allowed to rise from the bed.... I know of 30 drops of whisky given in a wine glassful of morphia by a night nurse, who herself was an opium eater!.... The matron...kept a baker's shop, and knew no more of real nursing than the poorest of the scrubbers. A patient recovering from a serious operation and under intensive care, came under the care of these night nurses and volunteer dressers, who often had been working and studying all day. I have sat up five nights in succession, from four a.m. till the staff nurse came on, relieving a gallant dresser, who took the first half of the night. Just imagine what chance a tracheotomy case would have under such conditions of nursing, unless the students volunteered.

The winds of change started blowing in 1856 when Miss Florence Nightingale returned to England at the end of the Crimean War. Revolution in nursing was in the air. When a grateful nation presented her with a monumental gift of £50,000 for her creation of a modern nursing system on the battle field she applied the fund in 1860 to inaugurate the Nightingale Training School for Nurses at St. Thomas' Hospital in London. The new era had indeed dawned, and the young Dr. Bell wrote to Miss Nightingale. She encouraged him to do something for nurses in Scotland. Years later he wrote: "In October of that year [1854] the Alma had been fought, and the Balaclava charge had roused the enthusiasm of the nation; Inkermann in November, [three bloody battles of the Crimean War] and cold, exposure, and disease all through that awful winter, had opened the eyes of the public to what the services needed for their sick and wounded were, and what Florence Nightingale and her staff tried so nobly to do. The impetus of that work and that woman gave the profession of nursing its first real start in the world, and by a reflected energy at last roused the hospital authorities all over the kingdom to action."

So—Joe Bell began by lecturing to the nurses; then he began giving "lab" classes. They followed him through various medical and surgical procedures; he taught them theory. When in 1871 he was appointed full surgeon to the Royal Infirmary and put in charge of the wards, it was no accident that the new system of nursing from St. Thomas's Hospital in London was adapted to the Infirmary. Joe Bell himself was instrumental in getting a Mrs. Taylor to act as instructress, a kind of Superintendent for the nurses. They were both interested in getting a "better class of women into the profession." Oddly enough, one of the first acts of the Infirmary Association at this time was to provide two quarts of ale to the nurses daily. "It was customary to give ale at mealtime to the Nightingale Nurses as probationers, with a view of lessening the risk of private recourse to simulants." After a debate "at which a committee of ladies" debated the virtues of a strong ale or Prestonpans beer, the brew drunk by the resident medical officers, the Prestonpans won out. Joe Bell, along with most of the doctors, decried the expense, and the new proviso was soon scotched, as it were.

There was a rapid succession of head nurses until Miss Elizabeth Anne Barclay, trained at St. Thomas's Hospital under the Nightingale Fund, was elected Lady Superintendent of Nurses at a salary of £100. Miss Barclay not only was St. Thomas-trained, but she also had gained experience in German war hospitals during the Franco-Prussian campaign.

He took his nurses round the wards with him on Sunday mornings, "and many yet recall with gratitude the valuable lessons then taught them which proved so helpful in their future work." So wrote Sir James Affleck at Bell's death. "It may be truly said that the development of modern nursing among us owes much to Dr. Bell—more indeed, than he has ever received credit for. Further, his interest in the welfare of nurses who came under his observation could be testified to by many who benefited by it. Dr. Bell became early connected with Queen Victoria's Jubilee Institute for Nurses, and was one of the most active members, as well as Chairman of the Committee, of the Scottish Branch."

On June 12, 1880, Florence Nightingale, writing to the Infirmary, speaks of Joe Bell "with the highest regards and most hearty thanks for all he has done so wisely and so well for the cause of Trained Nursing." A year earlier, when the new Infirmary finally was completed, Miss Nightingale, "who never lost her interest in the Royal Infirmary, gave practical help to those engaged in selecting the nursing staff." Joe Bell, along with Miss Angelique Lucille Pringle, a personal friend of Florence Nightingale and successor to Miss Barclay, did most of the work in Edinburgh. On the site of the George Watson School for Boys rose the New Florence

Nightingale home for nurses.

Because of his own work and the newly trained nurses, Joe Bell could say in 1892:

> The students of this generation know only of wards and beds perfect in cleanliness, even in luxuriousness of bright detail, of thoroughly educated and equipped women who as staff nurses, night nurses, and probationers, have each her own work, under efficient supervision and wisely arranged hours and methods.... No one is overworked, no patient is neglected, the poorest tramp has a chance of recovery certainly as good as the richest peer.... Now each ward has its own skilled trained nightnurse with a night superintendent to visit her once or twice during her vigil, and every serious operation... has its own special nurse, night and day, when needed.

Joe Bell, Florence Nightingale, and the new Nightingale method, especially under Miss Pringle, had come a long way. So successfully did he train the young ladies that "The visits of the Nurse were looked forward to, and her ministrations brought both bodily and spiritual comfort," wrote Mrs. Saxby. "Indeed it had been his experience to be greeted by an ailing [patient] with an expression of welcome for himself, but regret that he was not the nurse himself." So attuned did he become to the nurses' behavior and speech-patterns that years later, in his introduction to a volume of Sherlock Holmes stories, he said of the reading public: "Even the petty street-bred people are beginning, as the nurses say, to take notice [of mysteries].

More than just a footnote to Edinburgh Nursing history on the way to Nursing respectabilty and professionalism was Joe Bell's early and latter-day criticism. In addition to his early criticism of the inept, the lazy, and the inebriated who were on the wards as nurses in the '60s, he was even more unhappy with many of those who answered his call, the call of Florence Nightingale, and the call that rang in the editorials of the newspapers. While "he was interested in the movement for the higher education of nurses... he sometimes lost patience with what he called 'the young-lady craze for putting on a pretty uniform'."[35] The recruiting plan of the late '60s was working only too well. Unfortunately for the pretty faces, the lazy minds and the undedicated ones, Joe Bell found them out every time. In just a few years, the University (and some of the Infirmary staff) would have to deal with hopeful female medical candidates, and Joe Bell would have some of the same problems. As for the nurses, "I do not suppose," said Mrs. Saxby, "that the ladies who rushed into the ranks of sick nurses ever guessed how often their teacher felt inclined 'to laugh or say a sweer wird' over their inefficiency or their affectations." He knew what a good nurse could do. Just as Syme and Lister had Mrs. Porter, so Joe Bell had his own Head-Nurse, specially trained, and picked by him because of her powers of observation. "Don't be afraid to come to my Ward," he once told Mrs. Saxby, "you won't find one of your pet-aversions there. Nurse [Jeanie] Dickson is a real treasure, and worth a dozen of the new lady-nurses." Dr. C.E. Douglas, recalling Bell's career, also remembered Jeanie Dickson. "Joe Bell was so many-sided. The children, the women patients, the nurses all loved him for his kindness, his quick and ready sympathy, no one of them more so than she who knew him so well, his right hand all through his long service, his beloved staff nurse, Jeanie Dickson, on whose judgment he relied far more than on that of most of his residents." He did not like new, young nurses who wanted to "play nurse" any more than he liked the old alcoholics. If anything, he had more patience with the latter. Joe Bell wanted to see a spark of understanding; a willingness to learn, to observe; and he valued those who were devoted to their calling.

Most doctors, however, especially young surgeons, do not get so involved with nursing procedures—or the lack of them—as Dr. Joseph Bell. At the same time he began lecturing to the nurses and was trying to have the new system of nursing imported to Edinburgh from St. Thomas, he was beginning to develop his own practice. Many of the poorer parishioners of Free St. George's were among his earliest patients and remained so for years. He was ever grateful to them, treating many of them for token fees. It would never do, of course, to charge nothing. As he told Caird and Conan Doyle and other of his dressers, a good Edinburgh doctor must learn "Educated Scots," the Cowgate or Old Town Vernacular, and should realize that these were a proud people. Many a patient that he treated or operated on at the Infirmary became his patient too. He was gaining skill, confidence and patients. New Year's Eve of 1869 found him praising God for his dear wife and lovely children; loving healthy parents; and for the gift of life.

1869 was to be a momentous year. The Battle of the Sites was over. The new or Lauriston Site had been selected; his father, ever fighting for what he believed in, was pleased to contemplate a new hospital on a new site. The Governors of the Infirmary purchased over eleven acres of land contiguous to the George Watson Hospital. It was to be known as the Lauriston Site, and was described by Joe Bell as "the present palatial series of pavilions in Lauriston." It is doubly ironic that nearly all of the indefatigable biographers of Sir Arthur Conan Doyle were perplexed by the place name of the first "scene of the crime" in a Sherlock Holmes story. Enoch Drebber, redoubtable Mormon and formerly of Cleveland, Ohio by way of Salt Lake City, is found murdered at 3, Lauriston Gardens. Lauriston Gardens, said the biographers, did not exist. It sprung full-blown from Conan Doyle's imagination. Within the proverbial stone's throw from the New Infirmary were to be found Lauriston Gardens, Lauriston Place, Lauriston Lane, Lauriston Terrace, and Lauriston House. The new Infirmary at the Lauriston site will be completed, as we shall see, during Conan Doyle's second year of medical school.

Early in the year, almost without warning, Dr. James Syme suffered a stroke, and one can see from his own account that Joe Bell felt as though his world had gone into eclipse. He would continue quoting the medical and philosophical advice of his great teacher for the rest of his life. Meanwhile, he was asked by Syme to take over his class in Clinical Surgery, the summer session. He was to take the class of his mentor, his idol. He later recalls that he was too grief-stricken on first seeing the ailing Dr. Syme to worry too much about filling in for the Professor of Clinical Surgery, but Clinical Surgery was for him. He was more of a "demonstrator" than Syme, and established the pawky Scots humor and the Method of Observation from the beginning. He was learning, too, but he was in his element. So taken were they by their substitute that the class presented him with a special address, which was published two months later in the *Edinburgh Medical Journal* of September, 1869:

To Joseph Bell, M.D., F.R.C.S.

Edinburgh, 27th July 1869

We, the undersigned members of the class of Clinical Surgery in the University of Edinburgh, desire, before the close of the session, to express to you our appreciation of the manner in which that class has been conducted by you during the illness of Professor Syme.

We are mindful of the peculiarly difficult position you were called upon to occupy as the substitute of one whose world-wide reputation is indissolubly associated with his position as a teacher of Clinical Surgery.

It is pre-eminently necessary that he who would discharge with approbation the duties of this Chair, be possessed of that professional knowledge, dexterity, and courage, which the careful cultivation of high talent, combined with practical experience, can alone insure. From the constitution of this class, the capabilities of its teacher can be estimated by those who, like ourselves, are students, to a greater extent and with more accuracy than in any other in the University. We therefore feel it to be as much a pleasure, as it is certainly a duty, to assure you that you have obtained our admiration and esteem, as possessing, and that in eminent degree, those qualities which are so essential in a teacher of Clinical Surgery; and while, by the clear and forcible way in which your lectures were delivered, their subject-matter was impressed upon our memories, the hours spent in your class-room were rendered as pleasant as they have been profitable.—

(Signed by forty-three students.)

Syme had resigned officially on July 4, 1869, and in the same September issue of the *Journal*, following the address in fact, is the terse notice that "the Queen has been pleased to appoint Lister of Glasgow to be Regius Professor of Clinical Surgery."

Almost on the day that Dr. Syme resigned officially from his Chair of Clinical Surgery, July 4, 1869, Joe Bell received word from the Governors that he was appointed Assistant Surgeon to the Infirmary. The appointment came because of the great skill of Dr. Bell on the operating table and his manner and efficiency on the wards. A week later he was pleased to learn that he had been appointed Examiner to the Royal College of Surgeons. The young man admitted that to him there could be no higher position in medical circles than that of the Examiner of Surgeons. These men, after all, were ascertaining the skill of those who would hold the most "skillful, demanding, responsible jobs in all of Medicine." He little knew that he would hold that job for the rest of his life, and probably no doctor in the kingdom ever took a job with any more sense of awe and responsibility than Joe Bell took this one.

Toward the end of that summer term a son was born unto Edith and Joe Bell, and his name was, of course, Benjamin. It was Bastille Day, July 14, 1869. The parents were extremely happy, and the grandparents were overjoyed. Joe Bell, turning a new religious leaf, began taking the young Jean to Free St. George's on occasion.

His weekly "reviews" of the Sunday sermons (in his private Journal, of course) became more temperate. He was appointed Elder of St. George's Free Church toward the end of the year, just before his birthday. At 31 he was a man with a good-sized family, a growing number of students and patients, many titles and responsibilities, and "God's bounty all around."

Shortly before he was appointed Elder, he was informed by his friend and colleague, Dr.Patrick Heron Watson, that one Sophia Jex-Blake and six other women had been provisionally admitted to the University Medical School, despite "much ill feeling towards them." It was a new situation: women in the classrooms, wards and operating theatres occupied hitherto solely by men. Perhaps all Dr. Watsons like the ladies. In any case, Dr. Watson was all for admitting the new hopefuls; Joe Bell, far more of a traditionalist, would say "No" three years later when all instructors were officially queried about their willingness to admit the women, but he was one of but a few doctors who took time to suggest (as asked) a sound, alternate plan. As we shall see, he went on to teach the women, but he was aware that the University insisted on separate (not mixed) classes for the women. Admission to separate, or all-female classes, would entail a considerable reduction in the number of beds—already insufficient—available for the teaching of male students, since the regulations for the qualifying course of Clinical Surgery stipulated that the course must be given in a general hospital containing not less than eighty beds. Consequently, if eighty beds were taken away or set aside for the women, the efficiency of the Infirmary as a teaching center for the large male population would be greatly reduced. If both sexes were taught daily on the same wards (but, remember, not at the same time)—then the patients would be subjected to the role of guinea pigs. Dr. Bell's original solution was to train the women at

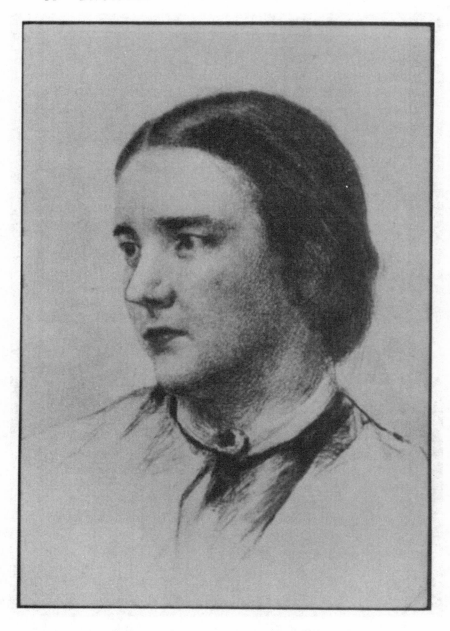

Sophia Jex-Blake, champion of women's rights, who tried to enter Harvard *and* Edinburgh med schools. Got six other ladies to register from 1870-1874.

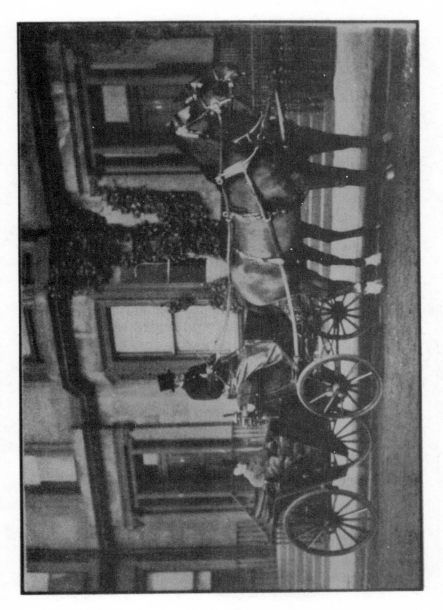

Making the morning rounds. Horses named Major & Minor by his children.

nearby Chalmers Hospital. We would do well to remember that Lord Stormonth-Darling called him the Peacemaker in this monumental battle. It was Joe Bell "who could usually see both sides of an argument."

The storm broke early in 1870. Abraham Lincoln incorrectly prophesied about Gettysburg: "The world will little note nor long remember what we say here, but it can never forget what they did here." The world, of course, has not forgotten the speech or the men. Most people have long since forgotten what Sophia Jex-Blake and a few doctors did in Edinburgh in 1870, but medical historians and all the advocates of Justice will never forget her.

Sophia Jex-Blake, in the perceptive view of one biographer, was "six years younger than her only sister and eight years younger than her only brother and suffered from all the disadvantages of an only child...." Disparity in age was enhanced by a greater disparity in disposition. Sophia did not "fit" anywhere.[36] She may not have fit anywhere, but she shook up the lives of most medical men in Scotland and the Kingdom in the '70s, and certainly impinged on Joe Bell's life, although he himself said *almost* nothing about it, as he was to do (and did) about many events of his busy life.

As a child she was described as "wilful, insubordinate, unladylike." Schools wouldn't keep her. Her older, evangelical parents didn't know what to do with her "mental excitability." Her father, a retired lawyer, wrote her: "Beware of excitability, your greatest enemy." He forbade her all the usual worldly pleasures, and Sophia felt the emptiness of her life. She heard of Queen's College, got permission to enroll: "Tried to speak to daddy last night," she wrote in her diary, but "he very impracticable, I after a while very undutiful. At last I went into hysterics, which frightened him dreadfully, poor old man. I shall certainly go. I think Michaelmass term begins 4th prox.... Poor old man, he is very loving and kind if not brilliant." She did so well at Queens's she was appointed to teach mathematics. Her father did not protest until he found she was to be paid for teaching. She would degrade herself, he insisted. Sophia logically asked why it was any more degrading for her to teach than for her schoolmaster-brother Tom (later to be headmaster at Rugby). Tom, her father said, was a) a man; and b) commanded a salary, after all, of £1,000. Oh, words too rashly said. She had him and he knew it.

Her immediate goal in life was a general reform of education. With that in mind, she took a post in Germany against the wishes of her parents, and upon returning home to Hastings, told her parents she was going to America to endeavor to reform education there. Her parents were terror-stricken. "I have such a prejudice against Americans," her mother wrote to a friend, "that I hardly ever will read a book describing American manners. I hate descriptions of low life."

In Boston she met Dr. Lucy Sewall, freedom fighter and Resident Physician to the New England Hospital for Women. Dr. Sewall mesmerized her. She met through Dr. Sewall scores of female doctors, professors and students. The two became firm friends, and the charming Dr. Sewall convinced her parents to let Sophia enter medical school in America. She had just applied to medical school in Boston in 1868 when she received word of her father's death. The "disobedient, headstrong, wilful" Sophia dropped everything to be with her mother. She tried to be a good nurse and comforter, but they both knew that propinquity was not for them. Through her brother Tom and a Josephine Butler, who had authored many "women's books" for Macmillan's, she decided to enter "the most prestigious medical school I know," the University of Edinburgh. In the spring of 1869 she was turned down, because the University after all was "not prepared to make temporary arrangements in the interests of one lady." The lady, with the super-abundant energy and intelligence, said to herself: "All right, if that's your game, let's try a new tactic," and in the summer of that year, she applied on behalf of herself and six other ladies who read of her plight in the *Scotsman*: Mrs. Isabel Thorne, who had lost a child in China, where she believed doctors treated men better than women; Edith Pechy, a vivacious lass of twenty-four who didn't know if she could "stand above the average man"; Matilda Chaplin Ayrton; Helen Evans Russel; Mary Anderson Marshall; and Emily Bovell Sturge. Sophia's on-the-spot analysis of Edith Pechy would do justice to Joe Bell or even Sherlock Holmes: "Strong, ready-handed, with great ability, resolution and judgment; great calmness and quiet of manner and action, and probably strength of feeling; good taste, good manner, very pleasant face; rather good feet and hands; considerable sense of humour, lots of energy and interest in things."

The red tape started to unwind during the July that Joe Bell was taking over Dr. Syme's class. The University Court that had denied a single female candidate entrance in the spring now turned the ball over, as it were, to the Senatus. After much deliberation the Senatus resolved that the seven could study medicine at the University. Sophia noted that "we all matriculated in the ordinary manner...paid the usual fee, and received the ordinary matriculation certificate which bore our names and declared that we were *Cives Academiae Edenenis*." Turner noted years later, "Thus in theory, if not in actual practice, admission was gained to classes within the University.

The seven women quietly went to classes in the fall of 1869. Sophia Jex-Blake was never happier, according to her biographer. The blow fell at the end of 1869-70 winter session. Many historians feel that most of the faculty and students, many members of the press, the average man, and many women sat back and smirked at the educational ambitions of the seven ladies, the first female undergraduates in any British university. Time and their naturally inferior minds would settle all. Then, lo! Their complacency was shattered. All the women passed and four with honors. Edith Pechey really ruined things by having the nerve and brains to win the coveted Hope Chemistry Examination. A series of events was set in motion by her achievement—events that would gravely affect the City of Edinburgh and much of the Empire for the rest of the century.

Professor Brown, greatly embarrassed by Miss Pechey's achievement and the sudden pressure put on him by a largely hostile and astounded faculty, did a lot of soul-searching. "He satisfied the claims of justice by awarding Edith Pechey one of the five bronze medals annually presented by the University to the five best students, and he declared the man immediately below her on the list to be the winner of the Scholarship on the grounds that the women, having been separately taught, could not rank as members of the class." While it was ironic that the scholarship money came from the exorbitant fees paid by the women in A. Crum Brown's class, it was a decision, whose "logic" would cost the women their medical degrees, because logically if Miss Pechey was not a "true member of the class" neither were any of the other women. If one were not a member of the class he (or she) could not present himself for the professional, final examination. Edith Pechey, from all accounts a quiet, lovely woman who wished to rock no boats, asked Sophia what to do. "We appeal," said Sophia, for the final certificate was essential. The Senatus, in one of the most illogical decisions in the history of education, declared, by a majority of one, that the women were entitled to the "ordinary certificate of attendance at the Chemistry Class of Edinburgh University," but that

Edith Pechey could not be the winner of the Hope Scholarship since she had not been a member of the class. "At this point in time," various slogans from the American stage come to mind: "You ain't seen nothin' yet; it's only the beginning"; and, from American sports: "Wait till next year."

Edith Pechey was no blue-stocking. The public and the Press were suddenly on her side, and the proponents of an all-male student body suddenly became alarmed. Public sentiment made the women more resolute. They had the Dean of the Medical College, Professor Balfour, and Professor Masson, of the Liberal Arts College, on their side. The opposition was led by Dr. Christison, Professor of Materia Medica and Therapeutics, and known as "Our Nestor" at the University. He was on every important committee at Edinburgh, and was also the Queen's doctor in Scotland. In addition Professor Christison was an expert toxicologist who had a European reputation. He was called in by the Crown for the most important criminal trials for poisoning and the like. Dear to the hearts of all readers of *The Sign of the Four* would be his lectures on curare, the deadly arrow poison of South American Indians. "When lecturing on curare... he used to come to the University a quarter of an hour before the class met to practise with the blowpipe [Shades of Tonga] so that during the lecture he might demonstrate how the natives made use of it. A target having been placed on one side of the classroom, he stepped down on the other side, inserted the arrow, took aim, and in a moment it was quivering in the bull's eye, and he returned to his desk amidst the rapturous applause of his class."[37] He was unalterably opposed to the women taking classes in medical school. He suddenly declared that he had invoked the opinion of "The Highest Lady in the Realm," and the Queen agreed with his own views on this subject. It was a bitter blow, especially since, as

Logan Turner surmises, it was "a statement possibly true but entirely unauthorized." Taking the bull by the horns, Professor Masson proposed (and Balfour seconded) that the women be admitted to regular classes. Dr. Christison rallied his forces to defeat the motion 58-47. It was a crushing defeat.

In 1870 Sophia learned the women could take classes with any professor (of the University) willing to teach them, and—most important—with any extra-academical lecturers whose courses were recognized by the University as qualifying for the degree of medicine. Thus in the fall of 1870 they approached the doors of the Royal Infirmary: As Logan Turner puts it, "The hospital with the crest bearing the motto of 'Patet omnibus,' ['It is clear to all'] turned them down, but to their everlasting credit, Drs. Peter David Handyside, Patrick Heron Watson, and Joe Bell, whose name appears almost nowhere in the fray, taught anatomy (Handyside) and surgery to the men and women together. George Balfour admitted both sexes to his class of systematic medicine. One of the few eyewitnesses of the day was Isabelle L. Jamieson, who was trained by Joe Bell as a nurse. Her daughter, Esme Gunn, a resident of Edinburgh, remembers her mother talking of Joe Bell training the nurses and training the women medical doctors. He had little patience with either when they let their minds wander. "Go home, go home," he would shout to the women students, "you don't know enough for me to be able to teach you anything." Miss Rose Upton, a nurse at the Infirmary in 1870, wrote to her sister that "Dr. Bell treated the women medical students like men. When he praised, he praised; when he chastised them, his voice cracked like a whip."

Thus the Battle of Attending Classes was won, but it became necessary to consider clinical instruction. All students (male, of course) applied for and were admitted to clinical instruction. The women applied and the

Committee of Managers of the Infirmary, a relatively liberal body, admitted them, especially since at least four extra-academical instructors were willing to give the women instruction. Dr. Christison realized that he had underestimated the enemy, and set about shoring up his defenses, while going on the offense. From this point on, the male undergraduates began to take part in the struggle. The women weren't their favorites. Their first step was to petition the Managers of the Infirmary to forbid the women access to the Wards. It was obvious to Dr. Christison and his cohorts that the authorities were not true champions of the women either.

    P.T. Barnum or the world's greatest Public Relations Specialists couldn't have set the stage more dramatically as classes began in October, 1870. In the Extra-Mural School the more serious students, and in 1870 that included all the women, started the winter term in October. All was quiet, and those working with Balfour, Bell, Handyside, and Watson were doing extremely well. The less industrious students entered on November 1 when the "full term" began officially. It was obvious that a concerted plan was afoot to embarrass the women. The young men jeered at the women, laughed when they started to speak, and, in general, engaged in puerile attempts to embarrass them. Matters came to a head in the middle of November at Surgeon's Hall, one of the centers of extra-academical training. The occasion was a competitive examination. Street rowdies were present and police conspicuously absent. Traffic was suspended for an hour. Sophia, telling her little group to stick together, led them to the Hall, past the dirt, garbage, and epithets hurled at them. For people whose minds were supposed to be smaller than men's, they seemed to pose a big threat. When they reached the huge iron gates they were slammed in their faces by a group of medical school students who stayed behind them "smoking and handing about whiskey bottles while they abused us in the foulest language I'd ever heard."

Throughout the examination there was noise and shouting outside, and some of the male medical students led sheep into Surgeon's Hall. After the examination Joe Bell and Dr. Handyside suggested that the young ladies depart singly by the back door. Sophia knew they were concerned about their safety, but she said dramatically, "I am sure there are enough gentlemen here to see that we get home unmolested." Unfortunately the protectors and attackers jeered each other, and the situation could get only worse, especially since the truculent students saw that most of the faculty were behind them. Edinburgh society lost its charm, said one of Sophia's biographers, because everyone took sides. While few approved the behavior of the male medical students many felt that "when women so far forget themselves to demand lives and careers of their own, they deserve much of what they got." In January, 1871, again the women were denied access to clinical instruction. One interesting result came from the campaign set up by Christison and his group in January, 1871. The women drew much public support because of the overwhelming opposition, and a Committee for Securing Complete Medical Education to Women in Edinburgh was formed. The Editor of the *Scotsman*, the Lord Provost of Edinburgh, and all the friendly members of the Medical Faculty were on it.

For the next two years Sophia, her little band of women, and the Committee tried to fight within the System. They took part in vigorous debates for the election of the Managers of the Infirmary. Sophia, in fact, was sued for slander after she had said that Dr. Christison's assistant used foul language to the women while intoxicated. When Christison demanded that she retract the word "intoxicated," Sophia gladly said that "If Dr. Christon prefers that I should say the assistant used foul language while sober, I will withdraw the word 'intoxicated'." The jury awarded the plaintiff one farthing. The committee succeeded in electing quite a few of their candidates. They insisted the women be allowed to go on the wards (this finally came about on a limited basis in the fall of 1872). The women insisted on being granted a medical degree, not a "certificate of proficiency." The degree, of course, was necessary in order to practice medicine. With the aid of the Committee, the Scottish, and, finally, the English press, the gallant Sophia took the legal battle all but to the House of Lords. They were defeated, but the question and the image of the woman doctor were now in the public eye. The female brain was no longer a laughing matter. Edinburgh made it a living issue.

From what the records and documents show, the gruff, capable, ever-efficient Dr. Patrick Heron Watson and Professor Masson had been their true champions. Joe Bell, cautious at first, taught them too. In the whole matter, as with the split in the church, and, years later (1897), the split in the management of the *Edinburgh Medical Journal*, he was the cool head (or one of them) that prevailed, or at least a head that kept the tempers of others at a reasonable level. Lord Stormonth-Darling recalls Sophia's storming the citadel in his beautiful eulogy (in the *EMJ*) of Joe Bell: "During all the long time [that I knew Joe Bell] there were questions from time to time arising—including the medical education of women—on which differences of opinion might quite well have arisen, yet I never knew a difference which could not be bridged over by moderation of view.... Dr. Joseph Bell... was indeed so wise a counsellor, had so level a head, and so perfect a temper, that it was impossible to take offense at anything he said. Moreover, he had a fund of humour which was not so much a fund as an inspiration." The battle of the female hopefuls was no laughing matter, however, and Joe Bell himself said almost nothing about it. He taught the young ladies, he allowed them on his ward in 1872-73, and he took over some of Dr. Watson's classes when that gentleman refused to allow Dr. Christison and others to alter his schedule too often. "There were giants in those days, but very combative and quarrelsome giants, and he [Dr. Syme] not infrequently found himself engaged in controversies which sometimes terminated in estrangement with men who were formerly his friends," said Old John Brown, who knew how seriously *most* doctors took things at Edinburgh.

As for Sophia Jex-Blake, she went on to get her M.D. at Berne; founded in 1877 a separate school of medicine for women. In 1876, meanwhile, the Medical Act (or Russell-Gurney Enabling Act) extending to the proper licensing bodies the power to grant qualifications for registration to *all* persons irrespective of sex, was passed. In 1878 women were allowed to enroll and take degrees at the University of London. In 1879, armed with her medical degree and a legal right to practise in Great Britain as a Licensiate of the King's and Queen's College of Physicians in Ireland, Sophia Jex-Blake returned to Edinburgh. Meanwhile, in Edinburgh, a city that had been bruised before London on this score, the Royal College of Physicians and Surgeons had resolved to admit women to their joint examinations. The Edinburgh Hospital for Women was created by her, and Leith Hospital, founded in 1848, opened its wards for the clinical instruction of women.

In 1870-71 Joe Bell was teaching Systematic Surgery to male and female students—separately, of course, most of the time. He was still giving special instruction to the nurses, and working hard at his relatively new job as Examiner of the Royal College of Surgeons. In 1871 he thought it time that some aspects of the examinations be updated. On October 20, 1871 he was appointed full surgeon to the Royal Infirmary. On October 23, 1871,

Joseph and Edith Bell and their three children moved to 20 Melville Place. He was now a full surgeon to the wards. One of his first acts was to see that the nurses got a broader and, at the same time, a more detailed look at the operation of the wards. He was also given a signal honor, usually granted older doctors, often to Chair-holding professors, to give the Introductory Address to the newly enrolled medical students for the Winter session of 1871. Joe Bell was but 33 at the time.

He was to deliver many an address in his life—he was, after all, witty, concise, and thoughtful, with a style and delivery shot through with grace. This, one of the earliest of his talks, however, says so much about his classical method of organization, his observation, his good sense, and his compassion that it is worth examining. He begins by comparing medical graduates with legal and clerical graduates. He ticks off statistics, but then notes that the doctor's forte should be something not too often taught well—medical ethics:

Our profession, above all others, involves personal relations. Lawyers may see only other lawyers, judges. A clergyman's intimate relations with his flock are too often very limited, but a physician is nothing unless he establishes the most intimate human dealings with his patient. It is not an easy task to hit the happy balance between kindness and sensibility; to be firm without being tyrannical; to be sympathizing, and yet escape the charge of humbug. Just think of the odds against us. When a man is ill he is almost certain to be cross. He may be bilious and have the gloomiest views of things—the past, the present and the future under one yellow cloud. If you are cheerful, you will be accused of want of sympathy; if you look doleful, he will think he is going to die.... Remember that to a sick man your visit is the one great event of the day; even a convalescent will put you only next in importance to his meals. So you must not be indifferent or careless.

Would that the medical Joe Bells of the world gave all the introductory addresses to young medical hopefuls.

Then, of all things, he tells them something that

probably few doctors would think of: "You should be amusing." He insisted on good humor on the wards. Then reverting to Biblical balance again, he advises: "Be kind and gentle, and you will have no need to try to appear sympathetic; be secret, and you will be trusted; be manly, and you will be treated as a man. Pretend sympathy, and you will be found out, sooner or later; gossip and fawn, and you will be treated as you deserve, as a sort of hermaphrodite, half monthly nurse, half tom-fool."

He provided the young students (still all male) with some inside information on medical ethics: "If called in haste to see another's patient, think, would you like him to do so for you. Answer 'yes,' if the case is urgent and real; 'No,' if it's a patient's fancy or folly.... Would that some of the grave, reverend seniors of our profession... spare an hour once a week to teach us Common Sense, the wisdom that too often has to be picked up... by many a slip and mistake." He then gives them some "instructive maxims" that are, on the surface, "elementary." (He refers over and over to various examples as "elementary.") First, "never look surprised at anything." He cited the example of the doctor who while bleeding a man in the bend of the arm, "wounded the brachial; a spout of arterial blood in a fine arch would have surprised any ordinary man, but not my friend, who caught as much as he wanted, bound up the wound, and sent the patient away with unshaken confidence in his skill." Then remembering things he learned from Dr. Syme: "Before stating your opinion of a case on a second visit, ascertain whether your previous directions have been complied with—i.e., do not compliment your patient on the excellent effect of your sleeping potions till you find he has taken it. Never ask the same question twice; this is very important, as, if you do, your patient will either be hurt at your inattention, or impressed by your stupidity."

He then becomes the fiery Joe Bell fighting for a noble

cause. In this case: preventive medicine—a field in which he seemed years ahead of most of his colleagues:

> Yet now a greater higher function than that of cure, is assuming a very high place in a medical man's duties. He must *prevent* disease, and then he need not have to sit with folded hands, or mournfully aver that he cannot *cure* till nature wills. What Jenner did for smallpox, some of you may do for measles and scarlet fever.... Ague has been banished from Scotland; we still have to get rid of cholera, typhus, and typhoid.... Believe me, the sum of preventible disease and death is enormous; and not till every marsh is drained, every city clean and wholesome, with deodorized [sic] sewage, and abundant cold water; not till every hospital ward is as sweet and wholesome as the air of the hills; not till food and warmth, air and water, are considered necessaries of life, need you complain the medical man has no work to do, or that your profession is a sinecure.

We are told there was applause, wild shouting, stamping of feet, more wild applause.

He continued, after "the longest period of great approbation," by reminding them that:

> Ours is not an easy profession. Others close their shop doors and leave, but for doctors be the fire and slippers never so comfortable, at the sound of that hated bell or knocker, your dreams of rest are rudely broken, and you are again in harness.... You will be sent for in haste by nervous ladies, when possibly you are ill and they are not. You will often be aggravated by finding yourselves requested by charitable ladies to see patients, they getting the credit for charity, you only the trouble of the visit.

(On the subject of being aroused, Bell, like Conan Doyle, was in the forefront of things scientific. As soon as telephones were available in Edinburgh, Dr. Bell had one installed, and the number 206B was forever after emblazoned on his stationery.)

He ends the address in a hushed tone, the firm high-pitched voice quavered. Today perhaps that ending seems melodramatic, "too much," saccharine, but Joe Bell, much like Henry Fielding in his battles against sham, pretence, and hypocrisy, meant every word he said and believed every word he said:

Few relations in life are more honourable and beautiful than those which exist between a sensible, manly, and skilful old doctor and his patients. He has seen the first of the children, the old people hope he will see the last of them. He has been present at every family gathering, sad or cheerful.... We cannot all be rich, or great; it does not fall to every one's lot... to be a Syme or a Simpson... but it is a noble profession, which offers to *all* the members a decent competence, respect in life, and regrets in death.

VII

"Bell The Busybody"—
Editor, Mourner, Master Surgeon, Master Teacher, Forensic Expert For the Crown

If ever the adage "If you've got something to do, give it to a busy man," applied to any man, it applied to Joe Bell. In 1873, because of his facile writing style; his devotion to medicine; his humor; and his busy-ness, he was asked to become editor of the *Edinburgh Medical Journal*, surely one of the world's leading medical magazines. In the van of those who asked him to serve was his friend and colleague Patrick Heron Watson. With almost no hesitation, Joe Bell accepted, and one may look until his eyes ache to find anything that he said about this gigantic task. He took over in 1873 and was to serve as editor for twenty-three years, stepping down in 1896.

He encouraged an international flavor when he took over. While the magazine for awhile may seem all Scotland, more and more notices, reviews and articles about the United States, the United Kingdom (including Canada) and the Continent appear. Joe Bell himself seemed remarkably aware of developments in American medicine. He revamped the Indexing system and greatly improved the quality and nature of the reviews. How he could possibly do all the other things in his life at the same time is amazing, but not until his death in 1911 did some of his unbelievable literary feats come to light. The editorial staff paid homage to him in the *EMJ* of November, 1911.

They noted that it was nearly forty years since he took over from Dr. George Balfour, and they (and Dr. Bell) recall the first number that he edited. "There were some twenty pages of type standing, no copy, and only ten days till the *Journal* was due. He set to work. He wrote articles and answered them, all under pseudonyms: and he accomplished the since unknown feat of publishing notices of *all* the books that had been sent in for review." He did not like to write editorials, but reviewed books, new medical programs and curricula, "and he was always willing to write obituaries. Within twenty-four hours of our request [after he left office] there would be dropped into our box a notice that would have taken most of us a week to prepare. He knew everybody, where he was born, something abut his family history, whom he married, the whole course of his professional life, and he had the happiest knack of referring to all these things in just the right number of well-chosen words."

Today the rift that developed "when the stream of medical journalism in Edinburgh for a time divided" is almost forgotten. It was right after Joe Bell stepped down from his post as editor—in 1897. Sides were chosen, tempers grew hot, and the various factions all turned to Joe Bell. Without hesitating, he "threw his support on the side of the *Scottish Medical and Surgical Journal*, of whose Directors' Board he was the first and only Chairman. When the stream flowed together again in 1908 no one rejoiced more, and no one was more responsible for the happy union than he, and he was unanimously chosen Chairman of the reconstructed Board." Just such a rift developed in his beloved United Free Church at nearly the same time, and we shall soon see the role he played in that.

So—in 1873 Joe Bell was now surgeon, private practitioner, teacher, editor, and devoted husband and father. During the year, William Earnest Henley put himself under the care of "the world's greatest doctor," Joseph Lister, and came to know Joe Bell. Bell found him an amazing man then, and called him "that talented genius" when referring to his creative and critical output. And just about the time that he was rejoicing over a third edition of his *Surgical Manual* coming out, the blow struck. He learned that Edith was ill—very ill. She was stricken with puerperal peritonitis, relatively common and certainly dreaded then, and "On November 9 [1874], at 8:05 p.m. Edith died."

No man could be more devoted, caring than Joe Bell. It is all he recorded in his Journal; he watched every physical change; he prayed more than ever, and he was a man who prayed much. He was greatly concerned about Edith's mother, who had been living with them ever since their marriage. "Edith died and was buried in the Dean Cemetery," a refrain that has a *leit-motif* quality in Dr. Bell's Journal. "The blow," he wrote, "is such a fearful one in its suddenness and intensity that I cannot realize it in the least, but I would *honestly* take it as sent by God for a good purpose in His infinite wisdom and love and would not rebel. Indeed I love my Saviour because he has been so good to my darling... and as I believe giving her an entrance into His kingdom." On her tombstone he had inscribed: "I thank my God upon every remembrance of you." It is superfluous to add to his lines. A week after his wife's death, he writes: "Lectured as usual. Boys very kind. All in mourning." His mother-in-law, the Honorable Mrs. Erskine Murray, died a few months later. She had been living with the Bells for nearly ten years. "I don't believe any mother-in-law ever was so good to, or so fond of, a son-in-law," he wrote. "I feel very left." One might be inclined to ask at this point if a man who cared so much for his mother-in-law were a saint or a stoic. Joe Bell was too loving and emotional to be a stoic, and he was too busy to shine halos.

Almost overnight, after Edith's death, the "jet black hair went iron-grey in three days of anguish," wrote his colleague Dr. C. E. Douglas. Nearly everyone who knew him and ever wrote about him commented on the sudden change. The free-flowing black became a stiff, bristly looking white. Miss Jane Sayer, a charming lady who knew Bell's daughter and still lives near her home in Kent, remembers Joe Bell's many visits to Cecil at Egerton House, "and when I was a young girl," she says, "I used to wonder if that shock of white hair was hard and bristly or soft. He sensed my perplexity, and asked what was troubling me. When I asked if I could run my hand through his hair to see if it was hard or soft, he laughed— very loud—bent down his head, and I felt it. Soft! Very soft it was." All who knew him say he was never quite the same man after Edith's death, and probably it was true, but he had great faith, a stern sense of duty, and three children to whom he was to become, if possible, more than just their father and mother. He threw himself into his work with renewed vigor, reacting to what he had once heard from Dr. Whyte about the "present vein of melancholy that shewed in Christian folk of the present day—so different from the sturdy faith and cheerfulness of early Christians." But Dr. Bell added: "Work is the key at present—work at your desk for the mind and work [outdoors] for the body." He concentrated more than ever on his own medical research (not too common even at the Infirmary) and the art of surgery. He was truly blessed in the devotion of Steers, Edith's nanny, to the children.

Joe Bell was an operator, a great one. He was in all probability better than Syme, better than Lister or Annandale, or any other contemporary, with the exception of the great-but-silent Patrick Heron Watson. While he was in the post-Listerian age, and the post-Simpson age, he would be operating many times in his life without anesthesia and when septicemia still plagued the hospitals. "Rapidity," writes a colleague, "was his keynote, swiftness in operating; 'getting the patient off the table and into bed' was his sound dictum; yet his work in plastic surgery [sic!], harelip, and cleft palate, work needing most careful and delicate handling, was a strong point with him; while in the management of urethral stricture he was perhaps the most dexterous on the staff."

He was praised, along with Annandale, by Syme and others for being one of the few young doctors who not only saw the great value and genius behind Lister's carbolic spray technique during operations, but one who used the spray. True, but Joe Bell was also one of the few doctors who not only saw, as Mr. Holmes would say, but observed what was actually happening with the blind devotion to the spray. In *The Surgical Side of the Royal Infirmary* he wrote:

The lightning-like speed of Liston and other great operators in the pre-chloroform days still lingered as a masterful tradition... but confidence in anaesthetics, and, still more, the early and devoted worship of the antiseptic fetish, tended to make an operation a very long business. By the time the spray engine was got in order, and the poor shattered limb was laved and scraped and shaved and bandaged, and any little vessel was tied, and douches of various kinds... were lavished on it... the surgeon was well into his second hour, and the patient, chilled, over-anaesthetised, and exhausted, was put to bed only to die in the early morning of the next day never having really had a decent pulse.

Corroborating and echoing Dr. Bell's words, Dr. F.H. Robarts wrote in 1969, "Even in Lister's day with a better control of infection the scope of operations had not altered much and the load and nature of surgical diseases was relatively unchanged."[38]

We have stressed the skillful, lightning-fast operators, but Charles Darwin in his autobiography recalls an operation that he saw while he was a medical student in 1828: "I attended on two occasions the operating theatre in the hospital... and saw two very bad

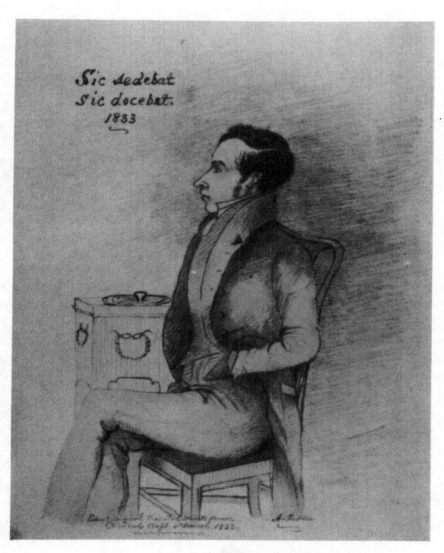

Student sketch of Dr. James Syme

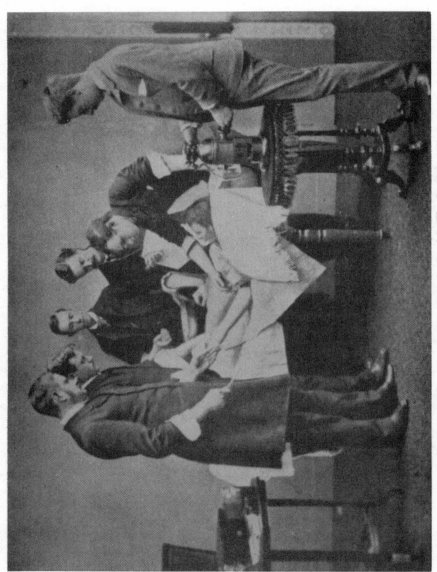

Baron Lister's steam spray called (by Doyle) "The Puffing Billy."

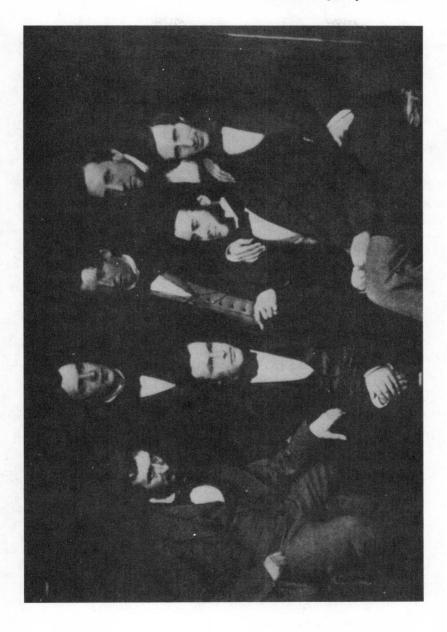

Baron Lister's circle of medical friends.

operations on one child, but I rushed away before they were completed. Nor did I ever attend again, for hardly any inducement could have been strong enough to make me do so.... The two cases fairly haunted me for many a long year."

What did Dr. Bell do about the problem? "My own invariable plan with cases of shock is to get the patient off the table as soon as possible, even though only a few stitches approximate a flap. Let me not be misunderstood. I am writing of primary amputations, for railway or factory accidents, where the shock is the chief factor in the case." Once again, it must be kept in mind that amputations, removal of the stone, and lithotomies formed the bulk of operations almost until the twentieth century, but in 1892, Dr. Bell wrote: "Cases are not refused, however, in the same manner-of-thumb way that used to prevail. I have seen cases sent home to die because a gland could be detected loose in an axilla. Such cases in 1892 are invariably allowed the chance of an operation." Before examining the acute medical eye and sense, the "years-ahead-of-his-time quality" about Joe Bell, it would be a shame not to look at his account of one of his own emergency operations. In the *Edinburgh Medical Journal*, March, 1879 he presented the following surgical case:

Double Primary Amputation of (Both) Thighs from Railway Smash
Rapid Recovery

G., a healthy-looking man, aged 27, but looking much older, while driving a horse near Granton, caught his foot on the edge of a rail at a point, fell, and both his legs were run over by several loaded wagons. A special engine was procured, his thighs tightly tied up, and he was sent up to hospital at once.

I was in hospital at the time, so with as little delay as possible he was placed on the operating table, and, the necessity for amputation being too evident, I obtained his leave to remove both his legs above the knee; but his pulse was very feeble, and he was intensely nervous, throwing his arms wildly about, panting for breath, and looking very ill, cold, and exhausted.

I determined that by great rapidity he might be got off the table alive, so operated in the following manner: Fixing the tourniquet firmly near both groins, I first amputated the right leg by Carden's method, and tied the femoral only, wrapped up the stump in a towel wrung out of carbolic solution 1-20, then took off the other limb by Mr. Spence's method,—it had been injured higher than the right, so that I could not save the condyles of the femur,—then tied the femoral there, and fixed it up with another towel, then returning to the first, I tied one or two large branches which spouted, and rolled it up again, then back to the left one, doing the same, and getting the tourniquet off both limbs. On going back to the right the surface was nearly dry and glazed, so, asking Dr. Maclaren, who assisted me, to stitch it up and insert a drainage tube, I did the same for the left, so rapidly that the patient was in his bed with his limbs dressed and bandaged in 24 1/2 minutes from the time he entered the hospital gate.

The strictest antiseptic precautions were observed, two engines being used to furnish spray. Of course, this great rapidity was due to the fact that everything was ready, the assistants all in hospital, admirably disciplined, and steam had been up in the spray engines. Shock was comparatively trivial; his temperature once, and only once, reached 100°. His stumps healed by first intention, and he was in the garden on the seventh day after the operation.... Had he been kept many minutes more on the table he would not have left it alive.

Perhaps even more uncanny were his observations and reservations of the contemporary medical scene and what he did to help remedy that which needed improvement. While Syme, Spence, and even Lister were praised for the swallow-tail coats or the vests that they wore while operating, Joe Bell, from his first-day swing around the wards with his nurses, told them, "I hold that hospital gangrene is in nearly every case caused by *dirt*, and dirt communicated to the patient by his *doctor* or his *nurse*. A great statesman once defined dirt as matter in a wrong place. Our view of dirt must be one that includes everything septic, all products of decomposition, everything that has a smell and many things that have not; and I hold that if we can eliminate these from our wards and bedrooms we will have no hospital gangrene." It was common practise for all surgeons to wear the same suit, the same coat, or the same white "butcher's jacket" or lab coat all day long—at every operation.

Joe Bell "washed up," taking particular care and time while doing so. He commented on the fact that probably even the faucet handles were unclean. Writes Dr. C.E. Douglas of Bell:

Before a thorough scrubbing, his preparation for an operation was to roll up his sleeves, displaying a vast amount of immaculate cuff. Looking back on those cuffs one sees in retrospect the white winged heralds of the dawn, of the armies of white-robed emissaries of the new dominant idea. They recall an episode, a type of the acute and practical observations of Dr. Bell. A delicate operation had been carried out with consummate art, the dissection of a parotid tumour.... A small vessel had been cut and the immaculate cuffs spotted. This is the only serious point, says Dr. Bell, indicating with his scalpel the spots of blood. The usual laughter from the benches followed, few noticing what the teacher meant, to wit, the pale complexion of the droplets, indicating the marked degree of anaemia. This in days when haematology as a science did not exist, was an important observation.[39]

Observation, observation. What a principle it was with him. He told the nurses, "Cultivate absolute accuracy in observation, and truthfulness in report.... For example, children suffering from diarrhoea [sic] of a wasting type sometimes take a strong fancy for old green-moulded cheese, and devour it with best effect. Is it possible that the germs in the cheese are able to devour in their turn the *bacilli tuberculosis*!!!" [Exclamation marks by Dr. Bell.] "Not a bad observation and deduction even for Sherlock Holmes some thirty-five years before Fleming and Penicillium notatum!" observes Dr. Robarts. Unlike Oscar Wilde, he did not agree that smoking was the "perfect pleasure" because it left one unsatisfied. He warned his students and those with slow circulation against tobacco.

"In 1873, Joseph Bell was among the first to chart accurately and faithfully surgical cases, noting the temperature change especially, after which the thermometer apparently came into general use," writes the most celebrated Scottish historian of medicine, John D. Comrie.[40] Getting back to the unclean hand faucets, in 1887 he seemed to be hinting at foot controls, and at the same time wondered if the wonderful steam engine that powered Lister's spray couldn't be harnessed or used to "sterilize" surgical instruments, although sterilization of instruments by steam was not dreamed of then. Finally, there is his keen observation on quite another subject in the *Surgical Side of the Royal Infirmary:* "Ovariotomy would require a paper to itself, hysterectomy to another; and what a warrior-poet-surgeon would be required to sing the epic of the wars of the tubes and the appendages! It is hard to believe that a woman has any other organs except those of generation, for all her woes [to the doctor] seem to centre in that interesting and lucrative region. As yet the male (probably because most operators are of the sterner sex) has escaped in a marvellous manner.... As yet, however, we have escaped castration for nervous symptoms, though it is threatened as a means of punishment."

In 1875, at the start of the new year, he vowed to a colleague that he would spend more time with his own children (he had always been close to them), and about this time began teaching *them* The Method. He also vowed to do something that he and Edith and Dr. Candlish had often talked about : the plight of the poor. Even when on holiday he often thought of the Edinburgh poor. From Perth, in the 1890s he wrote: "We are having the worst harvest weather I can remember, most of the crops still out and some not cut yet. Farmers will be hard put to it, and bread will be dear, I fear; coal also. I feel for the poor.... I would like to winter abroad, but I put it from me. It means so much for so many I like to help. Moderate work seems best for us on the whole." He was painfully aware of their horribly unsanitary living quarters; the aches and chills that seeped into their bones during the Edinburgh winters; and the general malnutrition. Thus, along with some fellow parishioners and some of the leading citizens of the City, he became one of the originators of the Longmore Hospital for Incurables, and, as the *Scotsman* said of him, "He discharged the duty of surgeon to that Institution up the close of his life. His interest in this work was of the keenest, and his regular visits were greatly appreciated by the sufferers whose burdens he lightened by his kindly sympathy and cheering words." Even more pertinent and perceptive, perhaps, were the words of a friend who saw Joe Bell at the Home: "His tenderness over the little maimed lives in the Cripples Home was womanly in its intuitive comprehension. But his warm sympathy never interfered with the cool decision necessary to his work, and many times the superficial observer thought he was indifferent to the torture of a patient seeing him pace with professional zeal, absorbed in the work of his hands." An extract from the minutes of the Home a week after his death also observed "We found him willing to consider the most trivial of details while no difficulty was ever beyond his power to solve." During his second week of visits to the Home he was elected Secretary-Treasurer to the Royal College of Surgeons.

Far removed from his work at the Longmore Hospital was Joe Bell's role as forensic expert for the Crown. When one is dealing with a quiet, modest man to begin with that's one thing, but when that man is called upon to perform top-secret investigations for the Crown, the silence can be profound. Obituaries of him, reports by his students, and even some scholarly books on the subject reveal little about Dr. Bell's role as a forensic expert.[41] This much is certain: In 1892-93, when he was being besieged by reporters as the model for Sherlock Holmes, he wrote to Mrs. Saxby: "Just see what the wretch from the *Pall Mall* has inviegled me into confessing.... However, I did not give the devil any secrets. Read what I said, and laugh as I do, at the persistence of your literary brethren." Among other things he told the reporter a little (very little) about his activities as a medical sleuth: "For twenty years or more, I have been engaged in the practice of medical jurisprudence for the Crown, but there is little I can tell you about it. It would not be fair to mention that which is the private knowledge of the Crown and those associated therewith...."[42]

The Boston *Medical and Surgical Journal* implied that many people knew of his forensic activities, but stated positively that "Bell served as assistant to Dr. Littlewood [sic] as official advisor to the British Crown in cases of medical jurisprudence."[43] He worked with one of the truly remarkable forensic experts of all time in Dr. Henry Littlejohn, equally well known as one of the first great Commissioners of Sanitation in the western world. So it would seem that Dr. Bell was one of the country's first consulting medical detectives, along with Dr. Littlejohn. One of his first well-known triumphs was the celebrated murder trial of Dr. Eugene Chantrelle, a suave, mutton-chopped Frenchman and one-time medical student.

Dr. Chantrelle, as he was called, was by all accounts a muscular handsome devil, who came to Edinburgh in 1866 as a teacher of languages. Before the end of 1867 he had seduced a fifteen-year old pupil, one Elizabeth (Lizzie) Dyer and had to marry her, but for nearly ten years theirs was the stormiest relationship imaginable. They exchanged passionate letters in the beginning of their relationship; she swore she gave herself only to him; he cursed her, abused her, and finally told her he was seducing the servants. Their letters ran from

"My dear Eugene,
    I accept you this day, as my lawful husband," and
"My dear Lizzie,
    I take you this day, as my lawful wife" to
"My dear Mama,
    I might have been sleeping for an hour or more, when I was awakened by several severe blows. I got one [from him] on the side of the head which knocked me stupid.... My jaw bone is out of place, my mouth inside skinned and festering and my face all swollen," etc.

He threatened her with a revolver, knives, and a final threat of poisoning her "so that not even the Edinburgh University faculty [sic] could detect his work." Almost ten years to the day, in October, 1877, the good doctor providentially insured his wife for over £1,000. Early one morning in December, less than three months later, the housemaid heard peculiar choking and moaning sounds coming from her mistress' bedroom. Rushing into the room, she found Mme. Chantrell unconscious. On the small French bedside table were a half-empty glass of lemonade, some orange segments, and some grapes. Keeping her wits, the maid called out for her master and then ran to fetch a doctor. Upon returning, she noticed the glass was now empty and the fruit gone, and her master making a hasty retreat from the window. The doctor immediately sent for Sir Henry Littlejohn, telling him he had a classic case of coal-gas poisoning. The great forensics man arrived with Dr. Joseph Bell. They both studied the bedroom, and had the wife taken immediately to the Royal Infirmary. She died within a few hours. On being told that his wife probably died of narcotic poisoning, Chantrelle told one and all that everyone knew they were having trouble with the gas in his wife's bedroom, but he was arraigned for murder.
    Bell and Littlejohn found evidence of poison

everywhere. There were many brownish spots on Mme. Chantrelle's pillow, a few on her nightgown, and analysis revealed that these spots contained opium in a solid form, along with minute traces of grape-seed fragments. The same combination was found in her alimentary canal. Dr. Bell learned from nearby chemists that Chantrelle had recently purchased at least thirty doses of opium.

M. Chantrelle loudly protested his innocence, always harking back to the smell of gas in the room. The maid insisted she smelled gas only upon her return from the doctor's. The gas company investigated and did indeed find a broken gaspipe behind a shutter outside the deceased woman's bedroom. The maid, who had heard and seen the arguments and blows over the years, felt that Chantrelle himself had ripped the pipe loose. Chantrelle objected that he didn't know the pipe existed. Suspicious, and doing what a good detective would do at that point, Dr. Bell located a gasfitter who remembered repairing the pipe for Dr. Chantrelle about a year earlier. He also remembered that Chantrelle was more than a little interested in the entire repair operation. With this development and Chantrelle's many letters revealing his sad financial condition, he was brought to trial. The four-day trial was the talk of Edinburgh. After deliberating only seventy minutes, the jury brought in a verdict of "Guilty as libelled."

On May 31, 1878, the dapper Frenchman was led to the scaffold. Z.M. Hamilton, who had heard such great things of Dr. Bell's classes that, even though not enrolled, he attended them regularly, gives an account of the condemned man's last mile: "The morning of the execution Chantrelle appeared on the scaffold beautifully dressed and smoking an expensive cigar. Dr. Littlejohn was there in accordance with his duty. Just before being pinioned, Chantrelle took off his hat, took a last puff on his cigar, and waving his hand to the police physician, cried out, 'Bye-bye, Littlejohn. Don't forget to give my compliments to Joe Bell. You both did a good job in bringing me to the scaffold'." Joe Bell said no more about this trial than he would say about at least three others in which it is known he was working for the Crown, and perhaps many others.

Indeed, years later in a controversy to be examined below, Adrian Conan Doyle, son of the author, rightfully said he could find Dr. Bell's name nowhere in the official accounts of the murder, but Sir Sydney Smith and two on-the-spot witnesses, Drs. Z.M. Hamilton and Douglas Guthrie, attest to Dr. Bell's involvement.

True to his word, he began to think more about the children's education, and if one can piece together various bits of information from Drs. Caird and Chiene, he invented something that sounds like The Game, featured in Kipling's *Kim*. It tested one's powers of observation and recall. He had also recently joined the Medico-chirurgical Society of Edinburgh and the Aesculapian Society, both, of course, medical societies. While he was certainly a "Clubable" man, one feels that he spent less and less time on them as the years went by. At the end of the year he was extremely pleased that his nurses shared with him a long letter they received from Florence Nightingale, who, in tone, style, attitude to God and self, sounds indeed much like Joe Bell:

New Years Eve of 1878
7 AM

Dear Nurses all, valiant and true

I bid you God speed & many, many happy New Years in our calling.
Let this be really a New Year: A Year of deliverances from all our faults & mistakes: (if you knew me, you would know how much I need deliverance from these:) a Year of pulling our Patients' through a year of

work such as angels might envy: a year of blessings for our Sick, of blessings for their Nurses: the "acceptable year of the Lord"—for us all.

And oh, remember that each one of those sick is a "temple of God," Let us not shame Him in his temple: that each one of those 'little ones' has an angel which "beholds the face of our Father in heaven." Let no bad news of us and our doings with each other be brought to our Father. He has given us a post: let Him find each one of us in it: true to everyone of his creatures as he is himself true to him.

Otherwise can there be any devotion to Nursing—any real care for the sick, any real love of the work? The place becomes a place of mere selfish occupation, under colour of "serving the sick": where each nurse may seek her own personal satisfactions, although in all the hurry & strain of hard work for others.

I know you *never* shirk your work: Yea even a hard working Nurse may not care about the sick. She may only care about her credit and her business.

I was going to say: What would I give to escape from my personal life & *lead* my Hospital life again & be one of you: But I perceive that would be doing what I have just said I would not do: seeking my own personal satisfaction.

So, *we* will remember—let who will forget it—the old "bundle of sticks"—

If we hang together in raising the Standard of Training & of Nursing, we can't be broken.

And let us at this time, the beginning of a New Year, "take stock" as it were of ourselves, our progress, & our work: I ask myself rather sadly, (but though I am an old woman, I don't mean to be beaten, I mean, please God Almighty, to reform yet)—I ask myself, I have been asking myself all night—*am* I keeping up to the motive that led me to choose this work? or do I look upon it merely as a thing to be got through?

Do I still think its a work to live & die for—a work to which God calls & called me?

King Harry the Fifth said, before he fought the battle of Agincourt with a few starving soldiers and won it, that if any man was afraid & wanted to go he should be welcome to go, & "crowns of convoy put into his purse."

"I would not die in that man's company
Who fears his fellowship to die with me."
I would not nurse in that one's company
Who fears her fellowship to nurse with me.

Am I daily pressing forward more & more to do the daily work for the good of others. Not for habit, self, of the glory of self—not merely because others are doing it & we *must* do it, like creatures in harness.

"Be not like dumb driven cattle,
"Be a hero in the strife"
I know a woman who said & who did it too: (She was the foundress of a great work) Be heroic in your *every day* & work: Your *every* day's

resolutions, even if you don't work up to them quite, you can do better every day.

We talk of rules:

This was her rule:

It was the rule of her life.

And if a heroine is one who does great things for the sake of another (no conceit, all humility in it—if she thinks herself a heroine, she is none—) & if any woman may be a heroine in small things & in daily life, just as much as in great things & on grand occasions, surely, any *Nurse* who has to do every day & to do & to do for others—any *Nurse*, may be a heroine.

Now hail to the Conqueror

O praise to the Lord

Our life is his Spirit

Our strength is His Word.

My very dear friends & fellow Nurses:

Let each one of all us Nurses be a

'heroine'

that is, let her do & be her very best in herself, in her common work with others, the common work in the 'Home,' the common work in the Infirmary—with everyone of the Patients—the common work with the others and assistants & all in doing their best.

Then if she does her very best, intending it to be better & better every day, till God raises it to the perfect work, she will be "heroic" in her daily work.

May we all be blessed in the New Year

May the New Year be blessed to all of us

    is the fervent prayer

        of your affectionate servant

                                        Florence Nightingale

VIII

Dr. Watson, Meet Sherlock Holmes: Dr. Bell, Meet Arthur Conan Doyle

Because of the unbelievable instant fame bestowed upon Sherlock Holmes and his creator, much of it was to rub off on Joe Bell once Conan Doyle let it be known (in May, 1892) that Dr. Bell was the model for the great detective. Their original meeting may have been a carbon copy actually of the classic Holmes-Watson meeting in the lab at St. Barts'. "For some reason which I have never made out," said Conan Doyle in his autobiography, "he singled me out of the drove of students who frequented his wards...." To get to Dr. Bell's beloved Ward XI in 1877 one had to pass through the little ante-room-laboratory in which Joe Bell, as keen a chemist as Holmes, performed his "little experiments" and lab tests.

In 1877, the new hospital was being built apace. There was much excitement, and in October, 1878, young Arthur Conan Doyle, a second year medical student, enrolled in Dr. Bell's Clinical Surgery Class at the Infirmary. As fate would have it, Joe Bell, who had been teaching systematic and operative surgery since the age of 26, reached the post of Senior Surgeon to the Infirmary in 1878, and at last eligible (and certainly able) to teach the subject of clinical surgery in friendly rivalry to the professor of that subject. Dr. Bell was one of the best-known of the Extra-Academical instructors, a rather peculiar phrase today, and one which will be clarified below. If young Arthur's grades didn't change drastically, his attitude did. Like nearly every student of clinical surgery, he was mesmerized by the method, the mind, and the style of the man in the operating theatre and the out-patient clinic.

In the "Surgical Side" Bell recalls how he was impressed by *his* classes with Syme, and from all accounts, especially since young Arthur was a far more romantically inclined sophomore, one can double Bell's feelings (expressed below) in spades, as it were, when it came to Doyle's views of him. Said Joe Bell of Syme:

Unless it was raining, the students attending Syme's wards might, if they chose, run down a steep flight of stairs, past one or two old houses...across a square of rough gravel surrounding a plot of measly grass, generally decorated by old broken iron bedsteads or decaying mattresses, to a low two-storied building in severely classical style [the old High School].... In the angle, dark and confined, of the lower floor of new Surgical Hospital admitting to the general surgical waiting rooms.... The large operating theatre, a really finely-proportioned and well-arranged building, with some small wards, house surgeon's rooms—extended beyond the main lines of the old High School, and formed part of a quaint old square, now nearly demolished, called Surgeon's Square.... I saw Dr. Syme daily for the greater part of his last fifteen years. His hospital life was on this wise,—two clinical lectures a week, operations two days more (perhaps three), a ward visit when he wished to see any special cases.

Driving down in his big yellow chariot, with footman, hammercloth, [a cloth covering the driver's seat or 'box'] and C-springs, with two big, rather slow and stately white or grey horses, he used to expect his house surgeon to meet him at the door and move upstairs with him to his little room, where he at once took up his post with his back to the fire and his hands under the flaps of his swallow-tail coat. In this little room he generally held a small *levee* of assistants, old friends, practitioners wanting to arrange a consultation, old pupils home on leave; and before his select class he examined each new and interesting case that could walk in.... Mr. Syme then and there made his diagnosis, which to us young ones seemed magical and intuitional.... Then if it was a lecture day, a tremendous rush of feet would be heard of the students racing to get the nearest seats in the large operating theatre.... Chairs in the arena were kept for colleagues or distinguished strangers; first row for dressers on duty; operating table in centre; Mr. Syme on a chair in left-centre. House surgeons a little behind, but nearer the door; instrument clerk with his well-stocked table under the big window. The four dressers on duty...march in (if possible in step), carrying a rude wicker basket, in which, covered by a rough red blanket, the patient peers up at the great amphitheatre crammed with faces. A brief description... and then the little, neat, tyro sees at once a master of his craft at work—no show, little elegance, but absolute certainty, ease and determination; rarely a word to an assistant—they should know their business.

He can not resist quoting Henley's words on the basket:

BEFORE

Behold me waiting—waiting for the knife
A little while, and at a leap I storm
The thick, sweet mystery of chloroform,
The drunken dark, the little death-in-life.
The gods are good to me:
    *   *   *   *
Here comes the basket? Thank you. I am ready.
But, gentlemen, my porters, life is brittle:
You carry Caesar and his fortunes—steady![44]

It is hard to know if it were consciously done, but Joe Bell followed after Syme along many lines. Early in his career (probably 1871), he bought two horses, both bays—always bays—called Major and Minor, names bestowed by the girls. They were hitched up to a barouche, a low, streamlined carriage, and when his practice started growing he employed a footman. Unlike his mentor, however, he eschewed the yellow exteriors and the rather garish C-springs.

The man had only Mr. Holmes as a peer in observation, and like Holmes he sorted out the important from the dross in "the lumber-room of the mind." The un-named medical-writer, who penned the bulk of Joe Bell's obituary for the *Edinburgh Medical Journal* also had his memories:

The large classes which Dr. Bell attracted testified to his capacity as a systematic teacher, but it was as a clinical teacher that Bell was in his element, and his theatre and his wards were always crowded. The interesting fact, to which so much attention since his death has been directed, that Conan Doyle from him drew the inspiration of Sherlock

Holmes has spread a far too wide impression that Bell was a superficial teacher. Nothing could be further from the truth. Behind those lightning diagnoses lay sound knowledge, and the students who followed him can look back on wise suggestions and prophetic hints which time has verified. The writer can remember today the *ipssissima verba* [exact words] were perhaps the outstanding feature of his teaching. Swinging rapidly along the corridor with his own peculiar gait, flapping the towel which he always carried, he dashed into the theatre, and, sitting down, spread the towel over his knees and began. Woe the out-patient clerk if the cases were not ready. There was great variety in surgical out-patients in those days. Eyes, skin, ear, and throat, or gynaecological cases—he was ready to tackle them all and to teach us something from each of them.

What was the magic of the man? What really happened in the operating theatre and the out-patient clinic. Dr. Clement Gunn, a classmate of Doyle's recalls:

We used to attend the Friday clinics held by Joseph Bell (the original of Sherlock Holmes) in the Royal Infirmary, in order to become acquainted with as many cases as possible. Bell's staff was so well organized that there was no loss of time; the patients all prepared in the side room, were run into the theatre with great speed, diagnosed and run out again. It was here that Conan Doyle, then an ordinary student like ourselves, observed, studied, and took notes, which he utilized thereafter in his stories. One young fellow, I remember, gave what was evidently a false name; but Joe Bell in writing the prescription calmly wrote down his real one and handed the paper to the patient. He blushed, looked sheepish, and departed. When he had gone, Joe said, 'I daresay you all noticed what I did then; it was obvious that John Smith was not his real name, but I saw the true name on his shirt-band.' Thus he trained us, his amateur "Watsons," in the habit of observation.[45]

How did he start the game, the Method? Speaking in his 'Rich Scots' he would pass around the class a vial filled with amber-colored liquid. In a voice of subdued humor ("we never knew how much he kept that sharp tongue in his cheek"), he would point out to each new class that "This, gentlemen, contains a most potent drug. It is extremely bitter to the taste. Now I wish to see how many of you have developed the Powers of Observation that God granted you. But sair, ye will say, it can be analyzed chemically. Aye, aye, but I want you to taste it—by smell and taste. What! You shrink back? As I don't ask anything of my students which I wouldn't do alone wi' myself, I will taste it before passing it around." He was obviously enjoying himself.

He would then dip a finger in the liquid, put his finger in his mouth, suck it, and then grimace. "Now you do likewise," and he would pass the liquid around. Each student would taste the harsh concoction, make a face, and pass the awful stuff to his neighbor. When the vial finally came back to him, Dr. Bell would look out over the pinched faces, and slowly start to chuckle. ("I believe that too was in 'Educated Edinburgh'," said Dr. Z.W. Hamilton.) "Gentlemen, gentlemen," he would coo, "I am deeply grieved to find that not one of you has developed his power of perception, the faculty of observation which I speak so much of, for if you had truly obsairved me, you would have seen that, while I placed my index finger in the awful brew, it was the middle finger—aye—which somehow found its way into my mouth."

That he observed with those eagle-like eyes, none doubted. Gunn continues, "One day a woman silently entered and, without speaking, handed to Dr. Bell a small vial, stoppered with a plug of soft paper, around which was wound some black thread. Joe immediately said, 'Well, ma'am, so your man's a tailor? And how long has he been ill?' The woman looked surprised and confirmed the information. When she had left, Joe remarked: 'It was quite evident that this woman herself was not the patient; she was too well. She wore a wedding ring, but was not dressed as a widow. The vial was plugged with some of those stoppers of paper on which tailors wind their threads when in use'." Dr. Bell's former student, Dr. J. Gordon Wilson, recounted an even more famous case of a woman patient—The Case of the Blistered Lip:

While Dr. Bell was seated at a table in the well of the amphitheatre with his interns and dressers, the patients were shown in by the outpatient clerk. On this occasion, awaiting his advice, was an old lady dressed in black and carrying over her arm a black bag which had seen service of many years. Bell gave her a quick glance and to our amazement said to the woman, 'Where is your cutty pipe? [a short-stemmed clay pipe] Her bag was on her left arm and instinctively she grasped it with her right hand.

This act did not pass unnoticed by Bell. 'Don't mind the students,' said Bell to the woman, much embarrassed, 'show me the pipe.'... She put her hand into her bag and produced an old short-stemmed, much used clay pipe. Bell quickly noticed the embarrassment of the old lady and whispered to his ward nurse, 'Let her lie down in the waiting room and see she does not faint.' As the patient was being led away, she whispered to the nurse, 'I began to feel faint.'

'Now,' said Bell, turning to the students, 'how did I know she had a cutty pipe?' No answer. 'Did you notice the ulcer on her lower lip and the glossy scar on her left cheek indicating a superficial burn? All marks of a short-stemmed clay pipe held close to the cheek while smoking—the characteristic attitude of the peasant woman smoking a clay pipe as she sits by her fireplace.'[46]

If this seems a pale imitation of Doyle's style, let us take the case of Arthur Conan Doyle himself. One of the most unperceptive statements he ever made was, "I couldn't see why in the world Dr. Bell chose me to be his out-patient clerk over all those others." Arthur, Arthur, how could you? Bell was always watching them. "Doyle was always making notes. He seemed to want to copy down every word I said. Many times after the patient departed my office, he would ask me to repeat my observations so that he would be certain he had them correctly.

"I recollect one time when a patient walked in and sat down. 'Good morning, Pat,' I said, for it was impossible not to see that he was an Irishman.

'Good morning, your honor,' replied my patient.

'Did you like your walk over the links today as you came in from the south side of town?' I asked.

'Yes,' said Pat. 'But the divil. Did your honor see me?'

"Well, Conan Doyle could not see that, absurdly

simple as it was. On a showery day, as that had been, the reddish clay at bare parts of the links adhere to the boot, but a tiny part is bound to remain. There is no such clay anywhere else around the town for miles.

"Once the patient was gone... Conan Doyle made me explain about the boots and clay, and he wrote my every word down in his little book."

In Doyle's own "The Five Orange Pips" Holmes tells his young client whom he has just met for the first time, "You have come up from the southwest," I see.

"Yes, from Horsham."

"That clay and chalk mixture which I see upon your toecaps is quite distinctive."

Or perhaps Doyle was remembering the patient who was stunned by Bell one day, a story that Hesketh Pearson heard from one of Doyle's classmates: "I learnt from another doctor who witnessed the incident that Bell flabbergasted one of his patients by saying: 'You came from Liberton [where Joe Bell's great grandfather went to farm and recuperate years before]. You drive two horses, one gray, one bay, you are probably employed by a brewery.' After the patient had gone Bell enlightened his pupils: 'I saw the clay from Liberton on the fellow's boots. He had gray hairs on one sleeve and bay hairs on the other. As for my final bit of deduction, you probably observed the face, especially the nose'."[47]

Doyle recalls he "had to array his [Bell's] out-patients, make simple notes of their cases, and then show them in, one by one, to the large room in which Bell sat in state, surrounded by his students. Then I had ample chance of studying his methods and of noticing that he often learned more of the patient by a few quick glances than I had done by my questions."

Doyle grew effusive with Harry How, a reporter for the Strand, in 1892: "Often I would have seventy or eighty [patients]. When everything was ready, I would show them in to Mr. Bell.... His intuitive powers were simply marvelous. Case No. 1 would step up.

" 'Cobbler I see.' Then he would turn to his students and point out to them that the inside of the knee of the man's trousers was worn. That was where the man had rested the lapstone—a peculiarity found only in cobblers'."

Dr. Harold E. Jones, a former student, recalls that Dr. Bell would insist that the students try his methods.

'What is the matter with this man, eh?' Then flashing a signal to one particular student with those piercing eyes, Dr. Bell would indicate he should pronounce the diagnosis. 'No, you mustn't touch him. Use your eyes, sir, use your ears, use your brain, your bump of perception, and use your powers of deduction.' The student, totally perplexed, stammered, 'Hip-joint disease, sir.' Dr. Bell would lean back in his chair, put those long delicate fingers together under his chin, and admonish the young man the same way he admonished the nurses and the female medical students: 'Hip—nothing! The man's limp is not from his hip but from his foot. Were you to observe closely, you would see there are slits, cut by a knife, in those parts of the shoes where the pressure of the shoe is greatest against the foot. The man is a sufferer from corns, gentlemen, and has no hip trouble at all. But he has not come here to be treated for corns, gentlemen. His trouble is of a much more serious nature. This is a case of chronic alcoholism, gentlemen. The rubicund nose, the puffed, bloated face, the bloodshot eyes, the tremulous hands and twitching face muscles, with the quick, pulsating temporal arteries, all show this. These deductions, gentlemen, must however be confirmed by absolute and concrete evidence. In this instance my diagnosis is confirmed by the fact of my seeing the neck of a whisky bottle protruding from the patient's right hand coat pocket....Never neglect to ratify your deductions.'[48]

Doyle himself recalls: "In one of his best cases he said to a civilian patient,

'Well, my man, you've served in the army.'
'Aye, Sir.'
'Not long discharged?'
'No, Sir.'
'A Highland regiment?'
'Aye, Sir.'
'A non-commissioned officer.'

'Aye, Sir.'
'Stationed at Barbados.'
'Aye, Sir.'
'You see, gentlemen,' he would explain, 'the man was a respectful man but did not remove his hat. They do not in the army, but he would have learned civilian ways had he been long discharged. He has an air of authority and he is obviously Scottish. As to Barbados, his complaint is elephantiasis, which is West Indian and not British.' To his audience of Watsons it all seemed very miraculous until it was explained, and then it became simple enough. It is no wonder that after the study of such a character I used and amplified his methods when in later life I tried to build up a scientific detective who solved cases on his own merits."[49]

Who can forget what is perhaps Doyle's best Sherlockian example of The Method. It has the same ring, timbre, cadence, and process as the case of the Man from Barbados. We find Holmes and Watson sitting with Mycroft Holmes in the bow window of Mycroft's famous Diogenes Club. The stout older brother and the detective observed two men stop opposite their window, down below upon Pall Mall. They ran their eyes over the smaller, darker man first.

"An old soldier," I perceive, said Sherlock.
"And very recently discharged," said the older brother.
"Served in India," I see.
"And a non-commissioned officer."
"Royal Artillery, I fancy," said Sherlock.
"And a widower."

The amazed Dr. Watson, thinking he was being "had" asked them to explain.

"Surely, said Sherlock Holmes, "it is not hard to see that a man with that bearing, expression of authority, and sun-baked skin is a soldier, is more than a private, and is not long from India."

To which the portly brother added: "That he has not left the service long is shown by his still wearing his ammunition boots as they are called."

Then Holmes noted: "He has not the cavalry stride,

yet he wore his hat on one side, as is shown by the lighter skin on that side of his brow. His weight is against his being a sapper. He is in the artillery."

Mycroft completed the analysis: "Then, of course, his complete mourning shows that he has lost someone very dear. The fact that he is doing his own shopping looks as though it were his wife."

Doyle did indeed take notes and he took them most carefully: he was learning from a master. If ever the legal tangle over the papers of Sir Arthur Conan Doyle is settled (it now threatens to out-distance Mr. Dickens' Jarndyce vs Jarndyce case), it may turn out that Sir Arthur the note taker was about as prolific as that other indefatigable Scottish compatriot of his, that other master note-taker and journal-keeper, James Boswell. Doyle learned about other things from his mentor, suggestions that would serve him in good stead as struggling doctor and as a writer: "When I took over his out-patient work he warned me that a knowledge of Scottish idioms was necessary and I, with the confidence of youth, declared that I had got it. On one of the first days an old man came who, in response to my question, declared that he had a 'bealin' in his 'oxter.' This fairly beat me, much to Bell's amusement. It seems that the words really mean an abscess in the arm-pit."

While, much like Sherlock Holmes, Dr. Bell could be (and was) kind to women and children, he was no "Patsy," no easy pushover. "Men admired and respected him as a helpful friend, or, if occasion arose, a worthy foe. He was never a man to trifle with, as the bagman found who pushed his way into the side room after a visit, an out-patient who disdained to mingle with the common herd at the clinic, and who found himself suddenly taken by the scruff of the neck and promptly ejected by the irate 'chief.' A Sherlock Holmes would have recognized at once his prototype. The piercing eye that took in everything, sizing up his man in an instant; the clear-cut mobile mouth; the beautiful hands, strong, supple, dexterous; the quick, alert step with its curious halt, in itself an honourable scar."[50] So wrote Dr. C.E. Douglas, another of Doyle's contemporaries.

Not all of Dr. Bell's lightning-quick diagnoses were played out in the great ampitheatre under gaslight. Dr. Charles Watson MacGillivray, writing about Old Harveians,[51] said, when he came to Dr. Bell:

> "Well do I remember the gasping astonishment of an outpatient to whom he suddenly remarked, 'Of course I know you are a beadle and ring the bells on Sundays at a church in Northumberland somewhere near the Tweed.'
>
> 'I'm all that,' said the man, 'but how do you know? I never told you.'
>
> " 'Ah,' said Bell, when the outpatient had left bewildered, 'of course, gentlemen, you all know about that as well as I did. What! You didn't make that out! Did you not notice the Northumbrian burr in his speech, too soft for the south of Northumberland? One only finds it near the Tweed. And then his hands. Did you not notice the callosities on them caused by the ropes? Also, this is Saturday, and when I asked him if he could not come back on Monday, he said he must be getting home to-night. Then I knew he had to ring the bells to-morrow. Quite easy, gentlemen, if you will only observe and put two and two together."

What of his wry humour, noted by Conan Doyle and so many others. He had tap-water wit, ready to pour out at any time, but he seemed—to those who did not know him well—quite serious. Edith, of whom we know really so little, but who knew of his great sense of humor, said, "People who hear him joking and laughing have no idea how tender-hearted he is. They can't believe that he feels things so seriously."[52] Vincent Starrett, probably the greatest Sherlockian scholar of them all, came across five of Dr. Bell's letters and was ecstatic about the find.[53] They were, he realized, "full of humor and common sense. Here and there it is possible to catch the dry inflections of the salty, deadpan lecturer haranguing his audience of young Watsons at the Royal Infirmary—or of the Sherlock

Holmes expressing a contemptuous opinion of an obnoxious visitor...."

All of Starrett's letters were from Joe Bell to Dr. Hugh Black, a co-minister when a young man at St. George's United Free Church. Dr. Bell was his physician and twenty years his senior. Starrett reminisced with Dr. Black's son, Robert K. Black, the well-known rare book dealer in Upper Montclair, New Jersey:

'Dad had several good stories about Bell's unorthodox method,' his son recalls. Here is one I have heard many times. One Saturday evening—the year would be perhaps 1902 or 1903—Dad was scheduled to preach the next morning and Mother thought he had a cold, although he assured her he was all right. She summoned Dr. Bell anyway, however, without telling Dad. He arrived promptly, without his medical bag or instruments, came into Dad's study and sat near him by the fire—and at once told him a very funny story. Dad laughted heartily. 'Ye'll no preach the morrow,' he said, and strode out. He knew by the sound of Dad's laugh that the cold was deep-seated, without having to poke in his throat and go through the 'Say Ah' rigmarole.

'Another story concerned a very proper titled lady who periodically suffered from delusions. Once she was certain she had gone blind. Bell perched himself at the foot of the bed and listened sympathetically to her complaint. Then quietly, without a word, he thumbed his nose at her. Her indignation was great. 'How dare you!' she cried. Bell may have lost a patient—I don't know—but he made it very clear to her that she was not blind.[54]

Starrett particularly liked the letter that Bell wrote about a lazy soul who suffered from inertia: "I have given him a prescription," Bell concludes, "tried to encourage him and advised *work*.

"I once gave a sturdy lazy beggar a certificate that he was suffering from *Inertia*. He got an allowance for some weeks from a society on the strength of it!"

Everyone, it seems, had his own famous Dr. Bell story. In his popular book, *Scouting for Boys,* Lord Baden-Powell recalls the patient who was brought into the ampitheatre, limping:

Dr. Bell asked one of the students the cause.

'I don't know, sir. I haven't asked him.'

The doctor replied, 'Well there is no need to ask him, you should see for yourself—he has injured his right knee—he is limping on that leg; he injured it by burning it in the fire; you see how his trouser is burnt away at the knee. This is Monday morning, yesterday was fine; Saturday was wet and muddy. The man's trousers are muddy all over. He had a fall in the mud on Saturday night.' Then, turning to the patient, he said, 'You drew your wages Saturday and got drunk, and in trying to get your clothes dry by the fire when you got home, you fell on the fire and burnt your knee—isn't that so!'

'Yes, sir,' replied the amazed man.[55]

We know that Doyle thought of him often, especially that fateful day when he first tried to dream up his detective. It seems Doyle's predecessor, Dr. A. L. Curor, Bell's dresser from 1871-1874, also remembered him:

It was the most thrilling and romantic point in our careers. I simply idolized Dr. Bell for his skill as a surgeon. I personally regarded him as a 'surgical sleuth,' but it was not until Doyle came along that the Sherlock Holmes idea was evolved. He [Doyle] saw, as I and others did, that Bell was a super-man [sic!] and conceived the idea of applying the surgeon's sense of detection to another purpose—fictional crime.[56]

J.W.B., a former student writing in the *Lancet* right after Joe Bell's death, recalled:

To many of us who studied in Edinburg in the later 'seventies' and early 'eighties' of the last century Dr. Joseph Bell was... one of the most attractive of the teachers of surgery.... His ward visit was always a breezy one. Carrying a towel in his hand, he passed rapidly from bed to bed, getting information.... [Later] we were told what had been the matter, when the operation had been, and were assured that the man or woman was getting along finely; very often, nearly always, the information was accompanied by a personal appeal for confirmation to the patient, and I remembered wondering if any of Bell's cases ever went wrong.

But the ward visit was nothing compared with the out-patient clinic: it was there that Bell amazed us all... with the rapidity of his diagnosis, with the brilliancy of some of his pieces of deductive reasoning, with the apparently irrelevant nature of some of the questions asked and more particularly with the confident statements made as to the calling habits, likes or dislikes, and place of birth of the [patients] who came into the theatre and passed out again, often in the briefest space of time. Some of us explained it on the hypothesis that Dr. Bell got a sight of the outpatient clerk's notebook; but the patients who came up late spoiled that supposition.

Despite Bell's reputation for punctuality and sticking to a schedule, Doyle as a dresser was not too flustered in ushering in the seventy or eighty patients a day.[57] He remembered other things, things that fixed themselves on his mind. He told Harry How: "All this [Bell's lightning-fast diagnoses] impressed me very much. He was continually before me—his sharp, piercing grey eyes, eagle nose and striking features. There he would sit in his chair with fingers together—he was very dexterous with his hands—and just look at the man or woman before him. He was most kind and painstaking with the students— a real good friend—and when I took my degree and went to Africa the remarkable individuality and discriminating tact of my old master made a deep and lasting impression on me, though I had not the faintest idea that it would one day lead me to forsake medicine for story writing."[58] In his autobiography Doyle noted: "I kept in touch with him for many years."

Doyle, like others, was impressed not only with his sense of humor, but also his manner with the patients. "He had a dry humour," he says in the Tribute, "and a remarkable command of the vernacular, into which he easily fell when addressing his patients." Mrs. Saxby and other colleagues remember not only his sense of humor, but that he had that one indispensable quality necessary to a true sense of humor: Joe Bell could laugh at himself. Since his students were nearly always impressed by his amazing string of correct diagnoses, occupation and origin of the patient, etc., they would nearly all ask him if he were ever wrong. He would usually laugh and say he was wrong on quite a few occasions, but his favorite story was the man with the puffed-up cheek. Bell observed the man, a bed-ridden patient, and said: "You are a bandsman."

"Aye, sir," replied the sick man.

"You see, gentlemen," the confident Dr. Bell told his students, "I am right. This man has paralysis of his cheek muscles, the result of too much blowing at wind instruments. All we need do now is confirm our theory."

Then turning to the patient, he asked, "What instrument do you play, my man?"

"The big drum," came the reply, and only the man with the aching cheek did not laugh uproariously.

Assuming that we can say Dr. Bell was definitely *a* model for Sherlock Holmes, the question has arisen whether Doyle ever used or pictured Bell himself in any of his stories. Curiously enough, one, never re-reprinted until 1979,[59] appeared in *Chambers Journal* of June 19, 1895, when Sherlock Holmes was no more, having gone over the famous—or infamous—Reichenbach Falls with the equally infamous Professor Moriarty. It was entitled "The Recollections of Captain Wilkie," the recollections of a con man. The teller of the tale is a young doctor, looking forward to "the gaities of Paris [after]. . . the dull routine of the hospital wards." His companion in a compartment on a train was Captain Wilkie, but our friend wanted to apply The Method, and see what conclusions he could come to about his neighbor. "I used rather to pride myself on being able to spot a man's trade or profession by a good look at his exterior. I had the advantage of studying under a Professor at Edinburgh who was a master of the art, and used to electrify both his patients and his clinical classes by long shots, sometimes at the most unlikely of pursuits, and never very far from the mark."[60]

In the adventures of the great detective himself, Holmes often leans back, "fingers pressed together." In

"The Yellow Face" we find "Holmes was turning the pipe
about his hand and staring at it in his peculiar pensive
way. He held it up and tapped on it with his long thin
forefinger as a professor might who was lecturing on a
bone."

Arthur Conan Doyle, who often "knocked against the
pricks of Fate" at Edinburgh University, was indeed
fortunate when Dr. Bell "singled [him]...out from the
drove of students who frequented his wards and made
[him] his out-patient clerk." He had decided to take
courses with an extra-academical teacher at Edinburgh
and he certainly profited thereby. He took an extra-
curricular course with Dr. Bell at the Infirmary. Since Joe
Bell was essentially an extra-curricular or extra-mural
teacher at the Infirmary, it would perhaps clarify things if
the extra-curricular idea were explained. Until 1840, the
University of Edinburgh recognized no other teaching but
its own. Dr. Bell's mentor, Dr. Syme, was the leader in the
movement to have the University recognize the
instruction at other universities, by other instructors.
Thus, in 1855, after a letter by Syme to the Town Council,
and after insistent petitions on his part, extra-mural
teaching was recognized. As of 1855 (when Dr. Bell had
just enrolled) University students could attend one-half
their classes extra-murally. Thus, not only could a
University of Edinburgh student pick up some credits in
London or Paris, but also he could take classes with the
more practical, well-known surgeons and medical men at
the adjacent Infirmary, one of international reputation.
Joe Bell, for example, could take course after course at the
Infirmary; Doyle, like many a student in the 1870s, not
only took courses from University professors, but often
took classes on the same subject from an extra-curricular
lecturer. As a result, "the number of extra-academical
lecturers increased and they lectured to large classes,
often greatly in excess of the numbers attending the

corresponding classes of the professors."[61]

There were various attempts to "organize" by the extra-mural teachers, principally because of the lack of classrooms. They were teaching all around Surgeon's Square, and the names of the "schools" indicated their locations: Surgeons' Hall, Nicholson Square School, Minto House School, the New (Bristo Street) School, and Park Place School. Of course, many of the greatest names were extra-academical lecturers: Balfour, Bell, Handyside, Littlejohn, Spense, Watson, etc. In the 1860s the class fee for each subject was £4.4s at the University and £3.5s in the extra-mural classes.[62] It is interesting to note that in 1879 practical instruction "at moderate fees" could be obtained at the Sick Children's Hospital, the Royal Maternity Hospital, the Royal Public Dispensary, the New Town Dispensary, and the Edinburgh Eye Infirmary.

Doyle himself paid £4.4s for his surgical classes with Dr. Bell at the Infirmary, and, according to his transcript, took his pharmacy classes at New Town Dispensary and a medical jurisprudence course at the College of Surgeons—all "extra-academical" courses.

Even though Arthur Conan Doyle took classes with and was in turn electrified by Dr. Joseph Bell, cakes and ale were still sold on Princes Street, and Charlotte Square,[63] Edinburgh. The instructor was becoming ever more the skillful surgeon and the pupil was going to have to start out on a practise of his own. The alchemy whose seed was sown, the catalytic reaction that took place, would take time germinating.

In 1879 the new Infirmary was completed amidst gala ceremonies. The Bells in general were pleased. On New Year's Eve, Joe Bell, following his wont, wrote in his Journal: "I would at the end of another year offer my gratitude for personal and family mercies and for the health and happiness God has given us all, and for the aid to me in my profession and class—and for the provision made for my father's age. For all his unnumbered mercies, God grant that my soul may prosper and that I may not forget my Saviour who gives all things." A colleague, John Chiene, who also alluded to the new Infirmary as the Lauriston Pavilion, was "pleased to see Joe Bell and his little family there," and "Dismal Jeemy Spence," who was opposed to the new, George Watson site, and who was never supposed to smile, was "exceedingly pleased to see Dr. Bell and his children."

Just as there were a host of Lauristons around the Infirmary, so were there many Watsons. Of Dr. Patrick Heron Watson we shall say more when Joe Bell, like his student-turned-mystery writer, awoke to find himself famous (1892) because of Sherlock Holmes. George Watson's Hospital was founded in 1741 by a merchant banker. It has flourished ever since, and is one of Edinburgh's most famous schools. George Square Ladies' College joined Watson's in 1974, and is now co-educational.

John Watson's School, another school as a possible, Infirmary site, and located just west of the Dean Cemetery, was founded in 1828 as a charitable institution for destitute and fatherless boys and girls. It later became a private fee-paying school, and because of the withdrawal of the government grant in 1975 was forced to close, the pupils being taken on by the Merchant Company Schools.

On September 26, just before classes were to start at the new Infirmary, Joe Bell wrote the first of several poems dealing with places he loved and some of the bitter-sweet qualities of life. Like Stevenson, he loved poems dealing with the hills of home, places that were in one's bones:

Glendoick

We know the land we love the best
  And there we cannot stay,
But also He that made our hearts
  Knows we are sad today.

He knows the homely love and grief,
  The tender parting pain,
The hidden ties that bind us here
  Where our long dead remain.

The gladness of the morning sun,
  The softness of the eve,
The pleasure of the autumn fields,
  That loving we must leave.

Yet if to each in God's good time,
  Is given his heart's desire,
Upon the happy hills our feet
  May wander and not tire.

The pleasant places that to us
  Seem best of all be given
And this old home we lose on Earth
  Be found our own new heaven.

He may have been an ardent admirer of Robert Browning, but his poetry stems from his firm faith, and seems far too sentimental and plain ever to be confused with Browning's. The significant thing about the poetry at this time is that he can start writing about the grief he had so long bottled up inside.

Almost at the same time that he was turning to poetry again, he was invited into the Lawn Tennis Club of Edinburgh, and became a member. According to Professor Caird, he not only became a member, but as in all else, he decided to take up and study the game scientifically. Every autumn from 1863, with the exception of the bout with diphtheria in 1864, saw him in the fields, after the birds and the hares, at Glendoick, or Gonogil or Corsock. Immediately upon his return from shooting in 1880, he had one of the great pleasures of his life—helping "Miss Nightingale" select additional nurses for the new Infirmary, and in February, 1881 he began lecturing to larger groups of nurses and on a more regular basis. If he was at all aware that a fourth edition of his *Manual of Operations* came out at the end of the year, he said nothing about it.

The girls had long been playing 'The Game' by 1880 (They, as well as their father, played it with young Benjamin Bell.)— "When the family traveled in a train," Mrs. Cecil Stisted recalled to Irving Wallace,[64] "he would promise the children a treat, and when we got out of the carriage he would tell us where all the other passengers in the car were from, where they were going, and something of their occupations and habits. All this without having spoken to them. When he verified his observations, we thought him a magician." According to Mrs. Stisted there was never a more unselfish father. "Jean and Cecil write every day when we are absent one from another, and I write always every day to both, often just a scrap, but they would be very much surprised, and think I was dead, if they did not get that scrap."[65]

In August of 1881 he wrote to Jean of the Queen's visit to Edinburgh and to his ward. As usual he was low-keyed, especially compared to the *Scotsman's* accounts, though he told her the papers would do a glorious job. The Scotsman trumpeted, "Thursday, August 25, 1881. The day of her Majesty's visit to the Royal Edinburgh Infirmary will go down as a red letter day in the history of this magnificent institution." It seems a torrential downpour was raging outside, while the Queen, absolutely fascinated by Dr. Bell's surgical cases and his explanations, spent most of the afternoon on Wards 10, 11

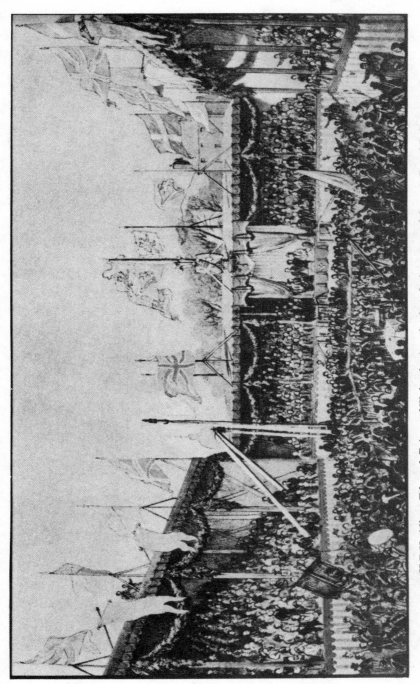

H.R.H. Albert Edward, Prince of Wales, laying the foundation stone of the new Royal Infirmary of Edinburgh, October 13, 1870.

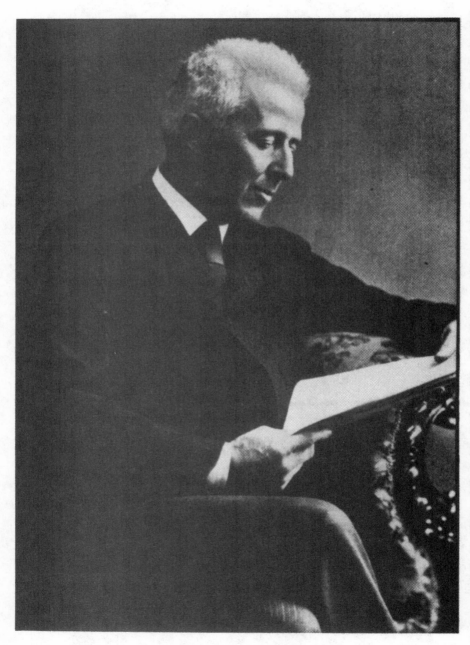

Joe Bell—aged 45

and 12, although only 10 and 11 had been "beautified for the Queen." The Queen was horrified by the post-operative wheezing sound coming from "a frail child's throat." The sound had been even worse when the girl was rushed to Joe Bell's ward. Holmes-like, Bell had ruled out the impossible, and realized that a minute foreign body was lodged in a ventricle of the trachea. He had performed a "lightning-fast tracheotomy and found a portion of the skin of goosebeery." The Queen was also much interested in the condition of a workman who "received somewhat serious injuries in preparation of the grand stand to be used in today's Review." Dr. Bell himself wrote the following account:

"My dearest Jean,
I am going to tell you a little about the Queen's visit though I dare say it will do much better in the papers. Well—we all managed—ladies, Provosts, I and two doctors met in the chapel where there was a throne and lots of chairs... but the Queen wanted to go just to the wards. The Provost said, 'This is Dr. Bell, your majesty, and she bowed and I bowed and then she walked into No. XI which was lovely with flowers because *we* (Nurse D and I) knew she was coming and she was so good and went out among the patients.... No. XI is now Victoria Ward."

He says nothing here about the Queen's being impressed by his courage and skill during the diphtheria crisis in 1864.

One of the most obscure events in Joe Bell's life took place in 1882: he applied for the Chair of Systematic Surgery in the University. One can only wonder if his colleagues (or students) urged him on, for he certainly did not seem overly ambitious at the time. No one, however, has ever said a word about it. In a musty, bound volume in the University Library can be found his entire presentation:

1. A letter to the Curator of the University of Edinburgh.
2. A list of his contributions to surgical literature.

3. A second letter to the Curator by the applicant.
4. Testimonials from thirteen representative teachers of Surgery and Hospital Surgeons.
5. Letters from nine representative provincial practitioners.
6. Letters from 387 medical practitioners, chiefly former students in Edinburgh.
7. Letters from 254 students of medicine attending Mr. Bell's clinics in the Royal Infirmary.[66]

Since Patrick Heron Watson was also applying for the position it seems unbelievable that neither he nor Joe Bell was the successful candidate (the ultimate winner was John Chiene, their competent classmate and colleague.) Dr. C.E. Douglas avows that Dr. Watson lost out probably because he "kept on through-out his career a general practice."[67] That would have eliminated Dr. Bell also, although several doctors hint that he started to specialize. Both defeated candidates were on hand to congratulate John Chiene, now Professor of Systematic Surgery.

On the heels of his not getting the appointment early in the year, his mother died in April. Like many men from happy homes and large families, Joe Bell said very little about his mother. One thing is for certain: the eagle nose and piercing eyes of Joe Bell came from her. "You will be sorry for us," he wrote to a friend, "in the loss of our good mother. What a mother she was!" His father was shaken by his wife's death, and sank rapidly. A year later he too died. While his son may have sounded a little Victorian when he wrote of his father's death, "My dear father has at last got his wish and found mother," he wrote a stirring tribute for the *Edinburgh Medical Journal,* concluding with: "[He] was, in the best and largest sense of the word, an accomplished physician, combining the practical and theoretical teachings of the older men with the minute and microscopic research of the more recent, harmonizing them as far as they admitted of harmony; receiving, though not, of course, always accepting, whatever had the promise of progress in science, and applying what he accepted to practical use in the treatment of disease.... His patients could and did rely on him as implicitly as his friends did in other relations in life. And he was what all truly good and great men are, single-eyed and simple—

Multis ille bonis flebilis occidit.
[He worked/fell for the many].

After the death of his parents and a dearly beloved aunt, Joe Bell felt he was eldest of the new old generation. "Now *we* are the old generation," he wrote. All his life he'd been a kind of second father and mother to his siblings, and now he was, at 46, the oldest of that "old" generation. After much study and deliberation, he took the newest generation—Jean, Cecil, and Benjamin, to their new home at 2 Melville Crescent in February of 1884, and one of the first things he did in the new house was to set up a small laboratory.

During the next two years, he spent a little more time at home, a little more time with his private practice. "Those living in Proximity to Melville Crescent," wrote the editor of the *Edinburgh Academy Chronicle*," might have set their watches by the passing of his carriage every morning at nine o'clock, no matter how busy and arduous the day, he would appear punctually to the minute at any appointment, professional or otherwise, which he had made."[68]

IX

Impediments to Early Retirement, Or The Game's Still Afoot: Another Job, Another Book, Jack The Ripper

On October 16, 1886, he must have really felt like the greybeard of the "old generation." He records in his Journal: "On October 16, 1886 I finally left the Staff of the Infirmary after... 15 years! Lord, comfort me I pray thee in my sadness in parting from my dear Wards and dear friends and nurses." While he was at the Infirmary much longer than fifteen years, he had been on the full-time staff that long. He was 49 years old. Sir William Turner, who was one of Dr. Bell's seniors when he was Demonstrator of Anatomy in the late 50s, observed: "The regulation which requires an ordinary surgeon to the Infirmary to demit [sic] office after a certain number of years of service, in the case of Joe Bell was a distinct loss to the school and to himself, as it removed from the list of teachers one who, from having been appointed when young on the surgical staff, was still in the plentitude of his experience and powers when the time for resignation was reached." Speaking of himself in the third person in "The Surgical Side," Dr. Bell says he can speak about the Infirmary with some authority, for "from the first day he entered its walls, a green and callow first-year student, to that day almost exactly thirty-two years later, when his term of office as senior surgeon ended, he never willingly spent a day in Edinburgh without entering its gates. From

17 to 49 is a large cantle of a working life, and equals one of
the three generations of men Nestor saw in his day; still, it
is to be hoped that the writer may not prove to be one of
Horace's typical old men, a

laudator temporis acti
Se puero, castigator censorque minorum.
[Praiser of the good old days but a censor of the present.]

It is a little difficult to know how to treat a 49-year-old
Surgeon-teacher at the height of his powers who has had
to resign. As some of the nurses observed in 1886, "On bad
days, he leaves the horses at home, and walks here [to the
Infirmary] faster than ever before. He is a walker." In
January of 1887 a large group of nurses, grateful for his
lectures "and for the kindly interest he had ever evinced in
their welfare," took up a subscription and presented him
with "a very handsome oak writing table and chair,
together with a brass writing set, a letter weight, and a
pair of solid silver candelabra. A deputation of nurses
from the Royal Infirmary, Longmore Hospital [the
Hospital for Incurables], the Royal Hospital for Sick
Children, and Prince Street Training Institution, made
the presentation at Mr. Bell's house."[69] In England,
Florence Nightingale, whose name was on the
subscription list, was chief contributor and organizer.

Meanwhile, on May 18, 1887 in the Hall of the Royal
College of Surgeons, Joe Bell, Senior Acting Surgeon to
the Royal Infirmary at the age of 49, was presented with
various testimonials, chief of which was a huge,
magnificent portrait of the good doctor himself. Dr.
Littlejohn, Convenor of the Presentation Committee,
summed up their feelings:

This is an auspicious occasion. Students, examiners, members of the
hospital staff, and college dignitaries, have met here to-day in this hall to
do honour to a gentleman, come of a good old stock, whose name is a
household word in the history of Surgery in Edinburgh, and who has

lately completed his term of service in the Royal Infirmary. That institution has always been singularly fortunate in its working staff, and never more so than at the present moment. Surgeons and physicians of eminence have ever been found ready to devote themselves to the discharge of the onerous and highly responsible duties attaching to their various posts, and it may be truly said, no institution has ever been more faithfully served. For thirty-one years Mr. Joseph Bell was connected with the Royal Infirmary, entering as dresser in 1856, and leaving as senior surgeon last year. Mr. Bell's whole career has been distinguished by the most honourable attention to his duties, whether as a teacher of systematic surgery in the Medical School, or as a teacher of clinical surgery in the Infirmary, whether as regards the patients committed to his charge, the nurses on his staff, or the students who thronged his class-room and wards. An accomplished and dexterous surgeon, he secured the confidence of his patients and the public. His teaching powers were freely devoted to the nursing establishment of the Infirmary, while to the students he endeared himself by the practical character of his teaching and his frank and sympathizing manner.[70]

It may have been a somewhat nostalgic time for the doctor, but no one had to feel sorry for the man. His talents and skills were in demand. First, he became Consulting Surgeon to the Royal Infirmary "upon the expiry of his term;" having been Secretary-Treasurer of the Royal College of Surgeons of Edinburgh for eleven years, he was elected president; the Royal Hospital for Sick Children, jumping at the chance, appointed him as their first surgeon on the children's ward, not, let it be said at the outset, just because he was available, but because nearly half the children's cases in the Infirmary were given or directed to him because of his way with them, his understanding of them, and the parents' love and respect for him. He was also busy finishing "a little monograph" (his words) for nurses. Joe Bell was, in essence, launching a second career. To relax just a little he began in the summer of the year visiting Mauricewood, a quiet, lovely estate at Milton Bridge, Midlothian—a few miles outside the city. His private practice was now thriving, and he was still editor of the *Journal*. Sherlock Holmes also made his appearance in the world in 1887, but if Dr. Bell happened to read *A Study in Scarlet* he certainly said nothing about it. With all of these events taking place in 1887, he also saw his *Notes on Surgery for Nurses,* dedicated to Florence Nightingale, published in September.

For once, he apparently read a review, and chuckled over it. In the *EMJ* for September, 1887, the reviewer seems crusty but fair:

> The dominant idea seems to have been not to teach nursing—that must be done in the wards—but to impart to the nurses an intelligent appreciation of the reasons, not only of their work, but of that part of the surgeon's in which they are frequently called upon to assist. Those who have studied Dr. Bell's other writings and especially his admirable little book upon Operative Surgery, will anticipate that at least in one important point, he thoroughly attains his end—he is perfectly clear. Dr. Bell's mode of teaching is similarly terse. It is calculated to dwell in the memory by its freedom from verbal diarrhoea. There is here and there, perhaps, a little constipation in the matter of conjunctions and definite articles.... The subjects of study are well chosen.

One of the first persons that he met on his new job was Miss Pauline Peters, who came to the Royal Hospital for Sick Children from the Infirmary in 1880 and became the Matron of Nurses. It was Miss Peters who arranged through the Infirmary's Matron of Nurses, Miss Pringle, to have the RHSC nurses attend Dr. Bell's lectures on "The Diseases of Women and Children" at the Infirmary. She also instituted the awarding of prizes to nurses and probationers for the best knowledge of Dr. Bell's lectures. The prizes took the practical form of a case of instruments.[71]

His new job: first surgeon on the children's wards of the Royal Hospital for Sick Children. As usual, he immersed himself in his work. In the early days of the Hospital there was no surgical treatment as such. The surgical ward was opened on November 1, 1887 when it was still at its original Meadowside location, and Dr. Bell

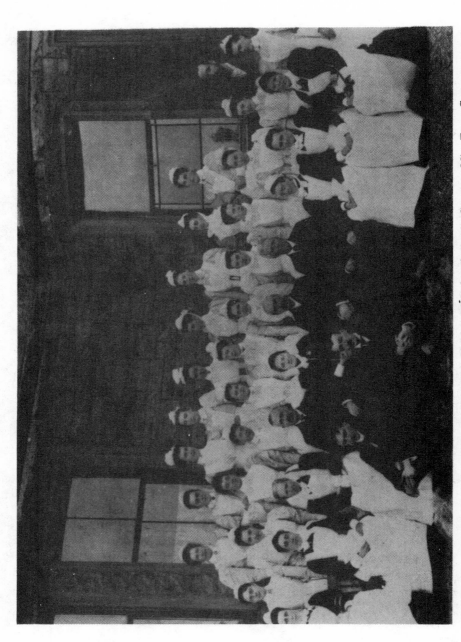

Staff picture: Royal Hospital for Sick Children, Edinburgh (1888). Courtesy Miss Esme Gunn.

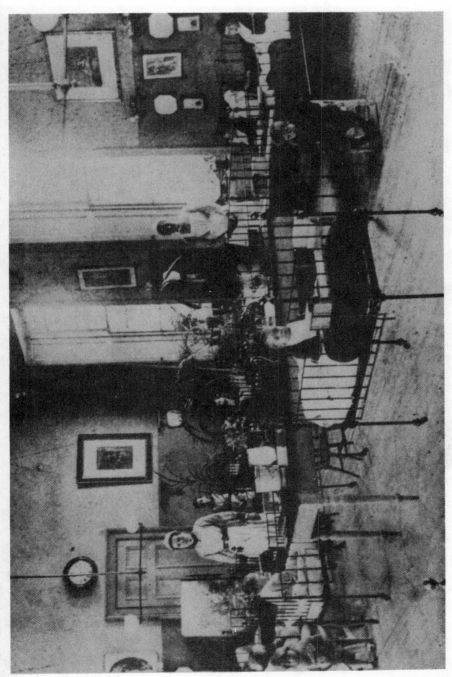

Ward at Royal Hospital for Sick Children, circa 1887.

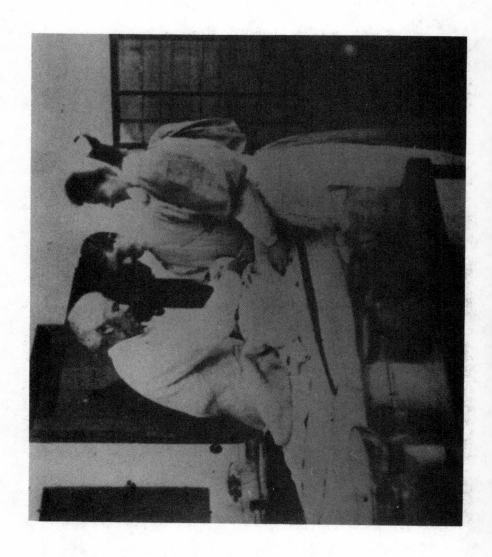

was put in charge. At first he had to use the "sewing room" for operations at Meadowside House, but at that location and at the new Sciennes Road Hospital, which was opened in 1892, "the surgical wards were filled to overflowing." Dr. Bell, in his monograph "Five Years' Survey in the Royal Hospital for Sick Children," noted:

> Street accidents of childhood; compound fractures from carriage, cart, and tram wheels; ruptured livers and intestines; falls from windows and stumbles on Salisbury Crag—are all swept into the waiting room of the Infirmary. Custom and easy access explain it, but the deformities of childhood—harelip, spina bifida, cleft palate, phimosis, and clubfoot—come to us in numbers, and hydrocele is very common. But the two classes of disease which choke the waiting-room of the Children's Hospital, and almost choke the beds, are joint disease and glandular swelling and suppuration. Had I four times the number of beds...I could fill them all in a week with cases of spinal disease and hip-joint disease.

In 1895 there were 1222 surgical cases handled by Dr. Joe Bell and his assistants, according to Dr. Guthrie.

His description of burn cases, peritonitis, and even severe injuries to the genital region are grim, but Child Neglect—Child Neglect Vintage 1890, incurred his wrath. One example is more than enough:

> W.F. *aet.* 5, was sent in from the country.... He had been brutally neglected and ill-used.... He weighs only 20 lbs. There is scarcely any subcutaneous fat on his body, or limbs. His hair is very thin and sparse...eczema on his head: His left forearm is ulcerated over the ulna, and there are several ulcers, apparently from frost-bites, on ears and fingers. On his right foot the large toe has sloughed off, leaving only the phalanx, which projects dry and black; the little toe has also disappeared.... This case was taken up by the excellent Society for the Protection of Children,[72] and the mother or stepmother...punished. The account given of his treatment was most revolting, as it was discovered he was kept in a cellar in the depth of winter, the floor of which was often actually covered with water, and that he had been systematically starved and neglected.

From the day he saw his first case of child neglect at the Infirmary, Joe Bell became the champion of those willing to cry out against it. For years, one surmises, many thought he was exaggerating the situation. As Dr. Comrie says, "He is ever to be held in grateful remembrance for his work as the first surgeon there."

Charles Dickens had come to Edinburgh in 1857, when Joe Bell was a young third-year medical student, and his heart was distressed by what he saw in the city. He saw desperately ill children lying in egg boxes. Speaking at a fund-raising dinner for the Sick Children's Hospital in Great Ormond Street, he reported:

> A little feeble, wan, sick child with his little wasted face, and his little hot...hands folded over his breast, and his little bright attentive eyes. I can see him now as I have seen him for several years looking steadily at us.... There he lay quite quiet, quite patient, saying never a word. He seldom cried, the mother said, he seldom complained; he lay there 'seemin' to wonder what it was a 'aboot.'

In *Our Mutual Friend* (1865), Dickens brought attention to the hospital for children thus: "We want to move Johnnie to a place where there are none but children; where the good doctors and nurses pass their lives with children, talk to none but children, touch none but children, comfort and cure none but children."

In 1873, Henley too was moved by the conditions for children at the Infirmary, and wrote his famous poem:

CHILDREN: PRIVATE WARD

> Here in this dim, double-bedded room,
> I play the father to a brace of boys,
> Ailing but apt for every sort of noise,
> Bedfast but brilliant yet with health and bloom.
> Roden, the Irishman is sieven past,
> Blue-eyed, snub-nosed, chubby, and fair of face.
> Willie's but six, and seems to like the place,
> A cheerful little collier to the last.
> They eat, and laugh, and sing, and fight all day;

At Night they sleep like dormice. See them play
At Operations: Roden, the Professor,
Saw, lectures, takes the artery up, and ties;
Willie, self-chloroformed with half-shut eyes,
Holding the limb and moaning—Case and dresser.

As F.H. Robarts reports, "It is well that 'Willie' seemed to like the place" for he was a patient for 846 days. 'Roden' was discharged after only 214 days...."[73]

At the same time we see the human side of Joe Bell a little clearer at the RHSC. "He was a great favorite of the little patients in the Children's Hospital. He kept a silver box full of chocolate pastilles which was produced for young visitors, and for older ones too. His family knew their way to it well, and he would liken them to 'the early Christians, who had all things in common.' "[74] From his own general observation and from his experience on children's wards, he could advise nurses in his new book:

Never deceive a child; tell it honestly that the dressing or movement you are going to make will hurt...but also that you will hurt it as little as possible, and it will help you loyally. Don't make favourites; children are much sharper than you think, and a quiet...child may soon get a sore heart...if you take less notice of it than of the more cheerful one in the next bed.

More than from any other hospital a children's hospital demands of its nurses that they show great kindness and consideration to the friends who bring in the child, and leave it, probably for the first time in its life, to the care of strangers.

In the now-celebrated passage about the cheese, Dr. Bell gently reminded the nurses:

You must always have the one great rule to guide you about sick children—that they don't cry or moan for fun, but because they are ill and in pain, or from a nameless weariness if not in actual pain. Healthy children may yell and scream as an evidence and result of original iniquity, but sick children don't.... If once you get a child's confidence and love it, it is marvelously loyal and utterly trustful.... Adults can read and amuse themselves, but a child's convalescence will often be much hastened by toys, cheering words, and...fun of the mildest type.

The stages in sick children are more rapid. Death is imminent before you are aware; yet, if staved off, recovery is like a miracle. They stand loss of blood very badly, and yet they remake blood every quickly.

Remember also that a child is nearly as reticent about its own symptoms as a horse or a dog. Watch what they eat or don't eat. For example, children suffering from diarrhoea of a wasting type sometimes take a strong fancy for old green-moulded cheese, and devour it with the best effect. Is it possible that the germs in the cheese are able to devour in their turn the bacillii tuberculosis!

In context, the repeated phrase about the mold certainly points up even more the fact that not much escaped the man.

As any nurse at the Infirmary or the new Surgical Ward of the RHSC could attest, there was the same sound advice, principles of sanitation and hygiene and the art of accurate observation in Dr. Bell's book on nursing as there was in the lectures and tours they took with him in the hospital. Some of the principles will seem like commonsense today, but many were not employed in the 1880s, and were formulated then by Dr. Bell, e.g., "In all cases when you have to dress or touch poisonous and putrid cases, just be careful first to see that you have no abraided cuticle, no rag-nail [sic], needle-prick, or raw blister; wash your hands in ammonia, or some such fluid that will nip a scratch; it will soon tell you if any exist, and if they are present, see that they are made safe."

Some of his admonitions would occur to the truly sensitive nurse; they would be violated by others:

Don't gossip about your last patient, and above all, don't tell blood-curdling stories of similar operations if you have a nervous surgical case. Don't get too familiar with the patients or the relatives.... Try if possible to see your doctor alone at least once a day. You may have to tell him, and he may have to tell you, things the patient need not know. But don't talk low or in whispers outside the door; and, above all, remember to give the patient a daily chance to see the doctor alone. She may have to tell him what she does not want a nurse to hear. She may even want to report some of your misdeeds.... Want of consideration in trifles—to hang an enema syringe to dry over a crucifix—will not be a way to win the heart of a high-church maiden. To turn the faithful old nurse out of her nursery will estrange, once and forever, the shy and ailing child.

He spends a good deal of time discussing the nurse in the home (home nurses were far more numerous than hospital nurses in 1887), and her relationship with the patient and the servants. His practical knowledge and good sense came through:

> You may want a thing brought up to your patient's room. Try to remember and note down...what you are likely to require, and let one journey do instead of many. If in winter, you have to keep up a fire, do not ring for coals when needed, but have a well-filled scuttle in the morning, and then you yourself, with old gloves on, wrap up pieces of coal in soft paper so that you can lift them out without either noise or dirt. Once show the servants that you are thinking of them and for them, and they will be your friends.... A nurse in a middle-class house with a few servants may sometimes be an intolerable burden. Airs and graces, meals at all odd hours to be carried up to her, constant ringing of bell for coals and hot water. If she expects the conveniences of a hospital in a private house, there will soon be friction.

As has been noted, he could be as rough and caustic with the nurses (or the women medical students) as he could be kind and considerate with them: "Never mind; keep your eyes open and *your mouth shut,* and you will learn something prompt.... Do not try to master the whole ward work in a week. In a large teaching hospital you will have lectures to attend, and much drudgery to go through before ever you have reached the privilege of dressing even an ulcer." At the same time, one knew he wanted to instill in all those who would have anything to do with the healing of human bodies, the same standards that drove and guided him. Above all, he was understanding of the human condition. Miss Esme Gunn, a life-long resident of Edinburgh, says, "My mother, Isabelle L. Jamieson, trained as a nurse at the Royal Hospital for Sick Children in the early 1890s.... She was a member of the operating theatre staff, and that is where she met Dr. Bell. The first time she appeared at one of his operations he asked her, 'My dear, is this your first operation?' When she answered in the affirmative, his kindly advice to her was: 'Look away while I put in the knife and then you may look as much as you like,' which showed his consideration for his nursing staff. He admired and respected competent nurses."[75]

Getting a little mellower, he ruminated over the history of nursing—describing the primitive, early days of the workhouse, the early hospital nurse:

> Often a by-word for cruelty and harshness [and who]...in the early Victorian era was part of a trade despised, but the trade now has a plethora of candidates for every vacant post....[Today] the age limit is well-defined: few are admitted before twenty-three, and practically none after thirty-five, so year after year hundreds of picked female lives are put under a training generally three years long. These women are trained to absolute unreasoning obedience [sic!], and invested with a graceful uniform, and rapidly acquire the *esprits-de-corps*, pride in their profession, and disciplined self-restraint which such a training is certain to endanger.... In a word, the profession of nursing is assuming a position not at all unlike, only a century or two behind, what evolution has made the profession of 'medicine.'

He then proceeded to give a lightning-like, capsulated version of the history of nursing in Edinburgh: It was a view of nursing unknown to most:

> A few years ago, in the novels which reflect the passing mood, and in journalistic literature generally, the trained nurse was, as a rule, all that was perfect; if she herself was not the heroine, she was at least the innocent self-sacrificing angel, who died after nursing a case of diphtheria, or was shot in the moment of victory. Bad men were made good, naughty women emulated her virtues, etc. Now the swing of the pendulum has gone the other way: the nurse is designing or even unkind. She is sometimes a minx, sometimes a new woman [sic], often a tool of the ruffian of the piece; and in the *Police News* we occasionally read, 'Hospital Nurse in the Dock,' 'The Nurse and her Lovers.' This change is not due to any deterioration in the quality of the real nurse, but to the fact that often designing women use the nurse's uniform and the nurse's name, both as a provocation and a disguise. Many untrained servants and even fast women masquerade in the nurse's uniform.... The Home

Nurse's salary will vary from £28 up to £40 a year, while a private nurse in good connexion [sic] can often make £100, or even more, and thus save for a rainy day.

He has a good deal of advice for the nurse in the country, and he was a practitioner who had many poor patients in the country: "The country nurse has trials of another kind.... Never say in one house what you see or hear in another; a small country place is full of tales, and each house knows far too much about its neighbour already.... Country people, till they know her, distrust the nurse, her uniform, her mania for cleanliness.... However, one case will soon tell another of her kindness, and in time her hands will be full enough."

Finally, he lets the nurses know that their bosses are the doctors—male *and* female. (His comments about the nurses' dealing with the women doctors have to be the first thoughts on the subject.) He begins, however, with the medical student (male) of the day: "However, remember the medical student of to-day is not the rowdy swaggerer of the early Victorian novels, but a highly-educated, hard-working, and courteous gentleman, who, as a rule, regards a probationer as a very unimportant and uninteresting person." While he may have caused a few lady-like (but hidden) smirks with his "gentlemanly qualities" of the young men, he was certainly realistic at the end of his statement. When he discusses the nurse's role with the practising physician, he tells them that the Edinburgh-trained, hospital-trained doctor may, in 1886, greatly differ from the doctor in the country district, "where the doctor left hospital before the new school of nursing was invented, and probably neither knows nor likes the new-fangled ways. All nurse's fine ideas of antiseptic treatment—sterilised towels and iodoform gauze—are met by cheerful disdain. He may even prefer to take his [patient's] temperature for himself, and he is apt to ignore the observations of the smart young probationer." Even so, says the doctor, even the highly trained hospital nurse and the veteran house surgeon can learn some things from the old practitioner. He concludes the doctor (male)—nurse relationship by warning that the newly trained nurses may become real threats to the doctors who hitherto had always lorded it over the nurses. When Joe Bell adds, "On their side let the nurses be obedient and gentle, and above all let them keep to their own duties," he too is echoing the old relationship.

While his discussion of the nurse-female doctor relationship may raise a few hackles today, it is based essentially on the dynamics being carried out before his eyes:

> Probably one of the most difficult of all relations is that of the trained nurse to the lady doctor. The nurse is probably older than her medical sister, for the nurse rarely finishes training till she is twenty-seven; a doctor may get her diploma at twenty-two. It is less easy for the nurse to obey one of her own than one of the opposite sex, and the lady doctor is very apt to stand upon her dignity. The safest solution of the difficulty is to fit the very young doctor with an old motherly experienced nurse, while the elderly lady doctor may be trusted to snub and dominate a young probationer.

Oddly enough, one of the first things that happened to him when he went to the RHSC was another visit from the Queen. She remembered him from his Infirmary days, and when she made a visit to the RHSC she made it a point to visit his surgical ward. He recorded, rather tersely, in his Journal on November 5, 1886: "Nov. 5, Queen visited.... I took her round. She was very pleasant—remembered me from Infirmary visit."

So well known was his skill and also his compassion at the RHSC that the modern reader could believe that all stories told about his days at the Children's Hospital were exaggerated or apocryphal. From the pen of one of his patients—Mrs. E. Winifred Binning, a vibrant 87-year old Edinburgh lady today—comes the following account, forwarded to the author by the gracious Mrs. P.M. Eaves-Williams, Archivist of the Edinburgh University Library:

A Memory of Dr. Joe Bell—Time May—June 1895.

I had had scarlet fever, following mumps, in the March-April of that year. We were living at Forest Hill, Muir of Ord, which had been lent to us for the winter, as my father was very ill, and he died there on 11 April. After the scarlet fever, I developed glands, probably tubercular, in my neck, and Dr. Pender Smith lanced the first, without any anesthetic. After my father's death, my mother would not go back to Dingwall, and I remember staying in Inverness with Dr. MacFadyen. I believe he told my mother—'If you want to keep that child you will take her at once to Dr. Joe Bell in Edinburgh.' So we came to Edinburgh. One afternoon we went for a drive in an open cab, and I was told we were going to see some little boys and girls who were ill, and that I was going to help to nurse them. I accepted this at its face value, and when we arrived at the Sick Childrens' Hospital—at that time at the end of Morningside Drive—I went in confidently. Sister met us and said to me 'I am sure you would like a little sleep, wouldn't you?' I was only three, and fell for it—I always did have a sleep in the afternoons. So I went off with Sister, and had my sleep, and wakened in a big ward with some dozen cots round the walls, and no Mother or Aunt Appie, Mother's eldest sister, to answer my agonised cries.

Next morning a young doctor came up the ward [Dr. Bell]—my cot was one of three across the end of the wall opposite the door, and backed by screens with windows behind—wrapped me in a blanket and carried me out of the ward. He took me behind a dark red curtain at the end of the corridor, and laid me on a table—no operating table or white tiles, or anything like that, probably less frightening for small child—and said they were going to give me something nice to smell and I was going to sleep. Chloroform mask applied, I obeyed orders, and Dr. Joe Bell lanced the second of the glands on the right side of my neck. Then each day came the dressings—one short tug at the cotton wool—one yell from me—and then clean dressing and bandage and peace for another day.

One day I was sitting up in my cot when Dr. Bell came round the ward with two lady doctors. He came to my cot and said, 'I want to show your neck to these two ladies.' Said I, 'You're not going to touch it?' Dr. Bell, 'No, Look, I'll put my hands behind my back and you can keep your eyes on them.' With that he turned his back on me, clasped his hands behind him, and stood like that until the ladies had inspected my neck. I don't remember if this happened during a 'dressing session' but I think it likely.

It is thanks to Dr. Bell and this sojourn in the 'Sick Kids' that I am able to write this now at the age of 76.

In the spring of 1888, he was "gratified" to see a sixth edition of the *Surgical Manual* and a second edition of the *Nurses Manual* published. He had worked hard in revising and enlarging the *Surgical Manual*. In the fall of the year, there occurred what was a relatively common accident in those days, but one which genuinely shook up the fatherly doctor. *The Scotsman* of October 10, 1888 reported the following: "Yesterday afternoon, Harry Kellarman, a coachman in the employment of Dr. Bell... met with an accident which might have terminated more seriously but for the prompt action of a lady whom he was driving at the time. While in Comistron Road his horse shied and bolted, and the coachman was thrown from his seat to the ground. Mrs. Bell [Cecil Bell, the younger daughter], the occupant of the carriage, at once got hold of the reins and brought the horse to a standstill. The driver was picked up unconscious and conveyed to the Royal Infirmary, where it was found he had sustained a fractured skull." In her interview with Irving Wallace many years later, Mrs. Cecil Bell Stisted indicated that her father inculcated unto the children, the Henry James admonition: Be One Upon Whom Nothing is Lost. They were to observe emergencies, observe methods, observe the cause of things—all to be able to act and when the time required. In his own Journal for October 9, 1888, Dr. Bell recorded: "Heard at night of accident to Harry and marvelous escape of the girl. Laus Deo." The next day he noted sadly that "Harry died at 11. Never conscious."

Late in 1888, according to the *Edinburgh Evening News*, Dr. Joseph Bell tried his hand in solving the biggest puzzle of them all: The identity of Jack the Ripper. It must be remembered, as Dr. Z.M. Hamilton reminded readers of the *Calgary Historical Bulletin,* Dr. Bell himself went on record, observing that "Dr. Littlejohn is the medical adviser, and he likes to have a second man with him... and it so happens that for more than 20 yrs we have done a great deal together, and it has come to be the regular thing for him to take me into cases with him." At the height of the Ripper hysteria Joe Bell received a report detailing all aspects of the case.[76]

The identity of "the greatest fiend of modern times" was never established. All evidence pointed to a person (women were not ruled out) possessed of no little anatomical skill; one who had a "thing" about prostitutes; and one who certainly was calculating and adroit, as evidenced by his uncanny stealth and elusiveness.

All of the murders took place in the Whitechapel Area of London's East End. From four to seven women were brutally slaughtered, dissected, and eviscerated by the murderer, probably starting in April of 1888 and ending at the very end of the year. Emma Elizabeth Smith, a widow, was the first of the official victims of the fiend. She was found in a Whitechapel gutter with her throat showing two jagged, parallel slashes that almost "carried" to the backbone. In early August Martha Turner, prostitute, was found dead on a tenement stoop, her body horribly mutilated. Three weeks later Anne Nichols, prostitute, "her body slit apart," was found in yet another Whitechapel gutter. On September 8 the body of Annie Chapman, 40-year old prostitute, was found in the back yard of a tenement, her head nearly severed and her organs laid out symmetrically around her—some change and jewelry at her feet. On September 30 there was a double murder. First, a man riding a pony evidently came across the Ripper as he was dissecting the body of 42-year old Elizabeth Stride. She had been attending a party. The murderer fled and seemed to disappear magically into the labyrinthian alleys of Whitechapel; later that night, the blood-drenched body of 43-year old Katherine Eddowes was found in a public square. The last and most horrible murder took place on November 8. Mary Jeanette Kelly, an attractive 24-year old prostitute, was found naked on her huge, old fashioned brass bed. Her throat had been cut through; her ears and nose sliced off; her organs had been removed and placed neatly around the body. On her pillow, above her twisted head—her bleeding heart. "The operator, according to Scotland Yard, must have been at least two hours over this hellish job. The madman [in a scene faithfully recreated by two recent movies][77] made a bonfire of some old newspapers, and by this dim, irreligious light, a scene was enacted which nothing witnessed by Dante, in his visit to the infernal regions, could have surpassed."

Along with the police, who nailed rubber strips to their shoes to promote silence as they walked in pairs around Whitechapel, Joe Bell was well aware that the killer used a long, razor-sharp knife; had a diabolic sense of the dramatic; and took unbelievable risks (everyone who owned a long-handled knife and knew anything of anatomy or wood-carving or slaughtering animals was suspect).

Some of the major suspects: a medical student with a pathological hatred of vice; a respectable English doctor whose body was found floating in the Thames after the last murder; a Polish barber named Koslowski, seen running from the Ripper murders; an American sailor; an insane Russian doctor; and, ironically, a real-life butcher.

Joe Bell was fascinated not only by the Ripper's letters to the London papers as well as the handwriting itself but also by the killer's maniacal delight in sending such things as human kidneys to the police. It is believed that, working out his own theory, he may have been instrumental in having the following story inserted on page 7 of the *Scotsman*:

Wed., Oct. 10, 1888

THE LONDON MURDERS

Detectives on a "New Scent"

The sudden disappearance of a man from a hotel in which he left a black bag, and is represented to have contained some articles of a compromising character. This man came to London from Scotland ten years ago. He is a duly qualified surgeon, but has lost his standing through dissipation. Since he began to slide the scale, his father has been in the habit of sending him remittances. The sums have been squandered among the class of women who have fallen victim to the murderer's knife, and on one occasion he was robbed of a case of surgical instruments by them. Since then, he has, it is said, harboured intense hatred against them.

According to the *Edinburgh Evening News*, Joe Bell spoke to a "journalist-friend" of Jack the Ripper murders, and related how he and another friend who liked solving deep problems, went about the unmasking of the fiendish murderer. "There were two us in the hunt, and when two men set out to find a golf ball in the rough, they expect to come across it where the straight line marked in their mind's eye to it[sic], from their original positions, crossed. In the same way, when two men set out to investigate a crime mystery, it is where their researches intersect that we have a result."[78]

He and his anonymous friend, taking into account all the Scotland Yard suspects and at least two additional suspects from Scotland, deduced the murderer; each wrote a name on a piece of paper; put the paper in an envelope; and then exchanged envelopes. Evidently both men had the same name (never revealed!). Dr. Bell immediately notified Scotland Yard. A week later, the murders came to an end. Was this coincidence? Did Dr. Bell and his unnamed friend have something to do with solving the case—or stopping the carnage? The answer will never be known, just as Jack the Ripper has never been positively identified. Sherlock Holmes, as a literary creation, was not yet a year old.

Less than five months later the forensics expert was

busy stuffing other kinds of envelops: his daughter Cecil was getting married to Charles Harcourt Stisted, a captain in The Royal Scots, and he was indeed the proud parent. On August 7, 1889, the couple was married by the Rev. John Thompson, Chaplain of the Earl of Roslin, at Roslin Chapel near Milton Bridge, a short walk (for the doctor) from Mauricewood. Four months earlier, in April, his only son, Benjamin, was commissioned directly into the Seaforth Highanders, Ross-Shire Buffs, the Duke of Albany's. Dr. Bell's only recorded comment, on the 9th of May, 1889: "Ben left to join the 72nd [Seaforth Highlanders] in Dublin."

In 1891, Dr. Bell was elected President of the Medico-Chirurgical Society. The Society, according to Dr. Ross, "was and still is an Edinburgh society whose members are physicians, surgeons, and general practitioners. They meet frequently in the Royal College of Surgeons, or the Royal College of Physicians, and there is a wide variety of subjects.... The society was a common meeting ground for all branches of the profession."

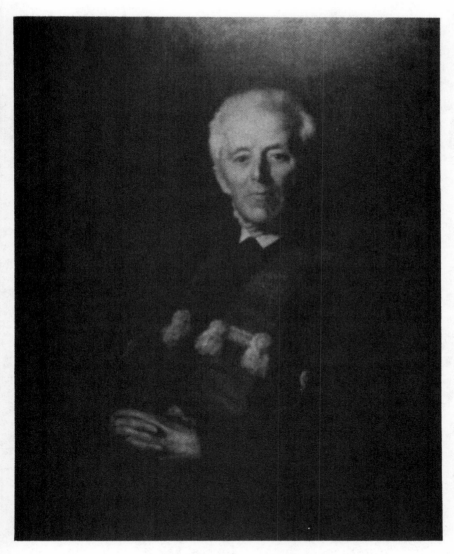

Portrait of Dr. Bell by Fides Watt (1896).

X

"I Read About You Everywhere":
Joe Bell, Model for Sherlock Holmes

In 1892, five years after the first Sherlock Holmes story appeared, Dr. Bell's busy-but-calm life was disrupted from a source so singular that, in a sense, his life was never to be the same again. Arthur Conan Doyle, now a full-fledged and full-time writer, was the celebrated author of one of the most famous characters ever drawn, Sherlock Holmes, and the journalists wanted to know all about him and his analytical detective.

The dam broke, as it were, in May of 1892 when Doyle, then living in South Norwood, wrote:

My dear Bell,

It is most certainly to you that I owe Sherlock Holmes, and though in the stories I have the advantage of being able to place [the detective] in all sorts of dramatic positions, I do not think that his analytical work is in the least an exaggeration of some effects which I have seen you produce in the out-patient ward. Round the centre of deduction and inference and observation which I have heard you inculcate, I have tried to build up a man who pushed the thing as far as it would go—further occasionally—and I am so glad that the result satisfied you, who are the critic with the most right to be severe."[79]

Doyle, apparently following up on a plot suggested by his old mentor, continued, "The deserter-cobbler is admirable. I wish I had a dozen more such cases. I am going to do 12 more Sherlock Holmes sketches next year so that I am insatiable for material...." He concludes by thanking him "very heartily for the 'tips'."

A month later—in June of 1892—Doyle penned yet another letter to his mentor—one that contained information about Holmes' character. His views here have seldom been mentioned or analyzed:

June 16, 1892

12 Tennison Road,
South Norwood.

My dear Dr. Bell,

Thank you very heartily for the photograph which I shall much value. Your permission will rejoice the cockles of Mr. Harry How's heart. It is an exceedingly characteristic and excellent likeness.

Holmes is as inhuman as a Babbage's Calculating Machine, and just about as likely to fall in love. The *Strand* insists on having a dozen more of his adventures for next year, and I am in great dread of letting him tail off. I have done the first one, however, of a new series and he is still going strong. I expect the book to come out about September. The Elections have demoralised the publishers.

With kindest regards,

Yours very truly

A. Conan Doyle.

The photo (of Dr. Bell) *was* cherished by Doyle, and reposed on his mantle.

Also late in 1892 Doyle sent Robert Louis Stevenson, whom he admired greatly, the first (and only) Sherlock Holmes stories that Stevenson would ever read. Stevenson had gone to Samoa for his health. Without having read Doyle's letter to Bell, of course, Stevenson wrote the following letter to Doyle in April of 1893:

Dear Sir:

You have taken many occasions to make yourself very agreeable to me, for which I might in decency have thanked you earlier. It is now my turn; and I hope you will allow me to offer my compliments on your very ingenious and very interesting adventures of Sherlock Holmes. That is the class of literature I like when I have the tooth-ache. As a matter of fact, it is pleurisy I was enjoying when I took the volume up; and it will interest you as a medical man to know that the cure was for the moment effectual. Only one thing troubles me: *can this be my old friend Joe Bell?*

Both Stevenson and Doyle's friend and collaborator, James Barrie, were University of Edinburgh students— non-medical—and they knew Joe Bell and his legendary reputation as a teacher. G.W. Balfour taught systematic medicine to Drs. Bell and Doyle, and in addition was Stevenson's uncle.

Harry How (his name is almost too good to be true), the intrepid reporter and feature writer for the *Strand,* went into action almost before Conan Doyle mentioned the letter for the first time; Mr. How was on Doyle's doorstep, seeking an interview, taking pictures, talking to neighbors. When Doyle told him that all the stories about Dr. Bell were true, How dashed off a letter to Edinburgh,[80] and Joe Bell answered most of his questions in a letter dated June 16, 1892. Even before Harry How dashed off his letter to Dr. Bell, Doyle wrote to him, mischievously warning him he might be deluged by "lunatic letters from Constant Readers who would request his assistance in rescuing maiden aunts from certain starvation in sealed attics at the hand of homicidal neighbors."[81] Mr. How had certainly worked fast. Dr. Bell seemed not at all reluctant to talk about Conan Doyle, The Method, or detective fiction. In fact, while he may have lost some privacy, he probably did not find the new-found fame nearly as opprobrious as Mrs. Saxby would have us believe. He once wrote to her: "The fiends of your profession [writers] won't let me alone, and I am haunted by a double whom you so hate, namely *Sherlock Holmes.*" As late as 1901 he wrote, "Why bother yourself about the cataract of drivel for which Conan Doyle is responsible? I am sure he never imagined such a heap of rubbish would fall on my head in consequence of his stories.... I hope folk that know me see another and better side to me than what Doyle saw." Before examining the Holmes-Bell similarities or lack of them, it would be more profitable and instructive at this point to see what Dr. Bell had to say about his former student and his relationship with the writer.

He told a reporter from the *Pall Mall Gazette*: "I always regarded him [Doyle] as one of the best students I ever had. He was exceedingly interested always upon anything connected with diagnosis, and was never tired of trying to discover those little details which one looks for."

The pages of *Harper's Weekly* carried more of the mentor's views of his famous pupil in February of 1894:[82]

> I should just like to say this about my friend Doyle's stories, that I believe they have inculcated in the general public a new source of interest. They make many a fellow who has before felt very little interest in his life and daily surroundings think that, after all, there may be much more in life if he keeps his eyes open than he had ever dreamed of in his philosophy. There is a problem, a whole game of chess, in many a little street incident or trifling occurrence if one once learns how to make the moves.

He had even more to say about The Method—it was closer to his heart. To the *Pall Mall Gazette* reporter, he said, "The great majority of people, of incidents, and of cases resemble each other in the main and larger features.... Most men have...a head, two arms, a nose, a mouth, and a certain number of teeth. It is the little **differences, themselves trifles, such as the droop of an** eyelid, or what not, which differentiates man."[83]

When asked for a specific example, Dr. Bell told him

what was surely one of Doyle's favorite stories. He told of the patient who walked into the room where Bell was instructing students. "He has been a soldier in a Highland regiment, and probably a bandsman." Dr. Bell pointed out the swagger in his walk, suggestive of the Piper, and from his shortness he had to be a bandsman. When asked about his station in life, the man said he was a cobbler and had never been in the Army in his life.

"This was rather a floorer, but being absolutely certain I was right, and seeing something was up, I did a pretty cool thing [sic]. I told two of the strongest clerks (or dressers) to remove the man to a side room.... I went and had him stripped, and I daresay your own acuteness [what a diplomatic way to speak to a reporter] has told you the sequel."

"I'm dashed if I do," said the Watson-like reporter—or words to that effect.

"Why," said Dr. Bell, "under the left breast I instantly detected a little blue 'D' branded on his skin. He was a deserter. That was how they used to mark them in the Crimean days." This is what Doyle meant by the deserter-cobbler case.

He elucidated on The Method in greater detail to 'Harry How and the *Strand* readers:

You ask me about the kind of teaching to which Mr. Conan Doyle has so kindly referred, when speaking of... Sherlock Holmes. Dr. Conan Doyle has, by his imaginative genius, made a great deal out of very little, and his warm remembrance of one of his old teachers has coloured the picture. In teaching the treatment of disease and accident, all careful teachers have first to show the student how to recognize accurately the case. The recognition depends in great measure on the accurate and rapid appreciation of small points in which the diseased differs from the healthy state. In fact, the student must be taught first to observe carefully. To interest him in this kind of work we teachers find it useful to show the student how much a trained use of the observation can discover in ordinary matters such as the previous history, nationality, and occupation of a patient.

The patient too is likely to be impressed by your ability to cure him in the future if he sees you at a glance know much of his past.

For instance, physiognomy helps you to nationality,[84] accent to district, and, to an educated ear, almost to county.[85] Nearly every handicraft writes its sign-manual on the hands. The scars of the miner differ from those of the quarryman.[86] The carpenter's callosities are not those of the mason.[87] The shoemaker and the tailor are quite different. The soldier and the sailor differ in gait—though last month I had to tell a man who was a soldier that he had been a sailor in his boyhood.[88]... The tattoo marks on hand or arm will tell their own tale as to voyages;[89] the ornaments on the watch chain of the successful settler will tell you where he made his money.[90] A New Zealand squatter will not wear a gold mohur, nor an engineer on an Indian railway a Maori stone.[91]

Nearly all of these "examples" are utilized in the various adventures of Sherlock Holmes.

In addition to The Method, Dr. Bell wrote about Doyle and Sherlock Holmes. He gladly wrote the introduction to the 1892 edition of *A Study in Scarlet*, and revealed an interest and knowledge of Doyle's works and other detective-fiction writers. He begins the introduction by blasting the tendency to gawk at and read about the upper classes in the scandal sheets. Doyle, he tells us, was trained to observe and appreciate minute detail, and thus he later saw, as a writer, how he could take the reader into his confidence and demonstrate Holmes' methods. Indeed, he says:

He created a shrewd, quick-sighted, inquisitive man, half doctor [sic], half virtuoso, with plenty of spare time, a retentive memory, and perhaps with the best gift of all—the power of unloading the mind of all burden of trying to remember unnecessary details.... He makes him explain to the good Watson the trivial, or apparently trivial, links in his chain of evidence. These are at once so obvious, when explained, and so easy, once you know them, that the ingenious reader at once feels, and says to himself, I could also do this; life is not so dull after all; I will keep my eyes open, and find out things.

A fair-sized and valuable book has lately been written on the one symptom, the pulse; to any one but a trained physician it seems as much an absurdity as is Sherlock Holmes' immortal treatise on the one hundred and fourteen [sic] varieties of tobacco ash.... The importance of the infinitely little is incalculable. Poison a well at Mecca with the cholera bacillus, and the holy water which the pilgrims carry off in their bottles will infect a continent, and the rags of the victims of the plague will terrify every seaport in Christendom.... Mere acuteness of the senses is not enough. Your Indian tracker will tell you that the footprint on the leaves was not a redskin's, but a paleface's, because it marked a shoeprint, but it needs an expert in shoe-leather to tell where the shoe is made. A sharp-eyed detective may notice the thumb-mark of a grimy or bloody hand on the velvet or the mirror, but it needs all the scientific knowledge of a Galton[92] to render the ridges and furrows of the stain visible and permanent, and then to identify by their sign-manual the suspected thief or murderer. Sherlock Holmes has the acute senses, and the special education and information that make these valuable; and he can afford to let us into the secrets of his method. But in addition to the creation of his hero, Dr. Conan Doyle... has proved himself a born story-teller. He has the wit to devise excellent plots, interesting complications; he tells them in honest Saxon-English with directness and pith; and, above all his other merits, his stories are absolutely free from padding.

Harking back to "the Well at Mecca" one should note that in *The Fabulous Originals*, Irving Wallace suggests that Conan Doyle's comment in his autobiography (1924) that Bell's plots for stories were impractical was not entirely accurate. The memory of the author had dimmed, Wallace suggested, for Doyle earlier had begged Dr. Bell to set aside ten minutes a day and think of plots. He also recalls a fairly well-known anecdote: "Dr. Bell suggested in 1892 that Holmes pit himself against a germ murderer, and hinted at knowledge of one such case. Doyle was quick to question if a bacteriological killer might not be too complex for the average reader."[93] Perhaps Dr. Bell's story of the water at Mecca contains the germ of that story. Remember also that the moralistic Conan Doyle felt the "Adventure of the Cardboard Box" (1893) was a shocker for which the world was not yet ready.

While none would begrudge the good doctor the privilege of writing introductions to the Sherlock Holmes stories, many objected to his being called "The Original Model of Sherlock Holmes." Since that debate was a long and hot one, and took place largely after Dr. Bell's death (1911) and even after Sir Arthur's death (1930)—let that serve as our coda. Leaving aside, then, the question of whether Joe Bell *was* the model, was he at all like Sherlock Holmes or Arthur Conan Doyle? How did they differ?

"The subtle, callous man-hunter tracking a criminal with cool and sleuth-hound persistency, had little, indeed, in common with the kind-hearted doctor, whose pity for a sinner was ever on the alert to help him out of the mire," wrote Mrs.Saxby just after Dr. Bell's death. Mrs. Cecil Stisted, the doctor's younger daughter, told Irving Wallace, "My father was altogether unlike Sherlock Holmes. The detective was hard and stern, while in striking contrast my father was gentle and kind." Even the great Sherlockian scholar, Dr. Douglas Guthrie of Edinburgh, felt that "after the lightning-like observation, analysis, and diagnosis," the comparison ended.[94] Holmes had some habits which were quite foreign to Joe Bell—his incredible untidyness, addiction to tobacco and even cocaine, music at strange hours and indoor revolver practice, all belonged to Baker Street and were unknown at Melville Crescent, Edinburgh.[95] The ladies and Dr. Guthrie come down pretty hard on Mr. Holmes. Actually Dr. Bell had a good many things in common with Sherlock Holmes, and perhaps just as many with Conan Doyle. Dr. Guthrie doesn't realize he is also describing the great detective, when he muses about Joe Bell: "A tall, stately man with aquiline features and alert expression." Pierre Nordan, the usually perceptive French biographer of Doyle and a man who had seen almost nothing about Joe Bell, felt that perhaps the world *needed* a model for Sherlock Holmes. He says of the Man-from-Barbados incident: "This sketch of Joseph Bell takes us straight back to Sherlock Holmes. It is too like Holmes to be true. Conan Doyle never describes Bell in a way that allows us to distinguish him from his fictitious character; it is as if Bell only existed for him as the function of a literary illusion." How little indeed he knew about Joe Bell (and one cannot blame him) when he goes on to say:

> Scientific prestige on the one hand and poetic realism on the other made it essential that a model for Sherlock Holmes be found *a pasteriori*, and that that model should be a man of science. We have very little idea what sort of man Joseph Bell really was, for Sherlock Holmes has blurred his outlines. While still a student, and before he had met Bell, the young Conan Doyle had probably begun inventing a rather vague imaginary character; then, when once he had fallen under the spell of his professor's personality, he found it intervening and filling out the details of his fictitious creation.[96]

Like Sherlock Holmes, all kinds of people came to Dr. Bell when they were in trouble, and not only for medical ailments. He inspired confidence, he was a soother. Some of the stories of his soothing powers border on the weird, but certainly not the supernatural or "spiritual." After his death, the Board of the Hospital for Incurables noted, "No difficulty was ever beyond his power to solve," and like Sherlock Holmes, when advising a patient or friend, he was, according to his protege, Dr. Caird: "Brief, lucid, almost epigrammatic in the use of words."

Like the great detective, he was, according to students, fascinated by "the technique" of boxing; he played hailes [not available to Mr. Holmes], cricket and football. Toward the end of his life, in fact, "he would spend more and more Saturday afternoons at Raeburn Place watching cricket."[97] While he may not have carved out the Queen's initials in the wall (hardly fitting for an Edinburgh physician), he spent years with the Artillery at Granton; went shooting in the fall for game at Glendoick or Glenogil or Pearse or Corsock, and when answering one of Mrs. Saxby's questions from a rather gushy Victorian questionaire-game, he said his "special weakness" was grouse shooting in September. Like Mr. Holmes, Joe Bell, a student recalls, had an eye "so keen he could spot the species of any bird on the wing." Both men could spend delightful hours over test tubes and retorts. Both men had their own observations on the police. What Holmes thought of Scotland Yard is fairly well-known; Bell's views are hardly known at all. He told a *Pall Mall Gazette* reporter that there was little special incentive for the special training of police, a serious error in Dr. Bell's opinion. "The fatal mistake which the ordinary policeman make is this, that he gets his theory first, and then makes the facts fit it, instead of getting his facts first and making all his little observations and deductions until he is driven irresistibly by them into an elucidation in a direction he may never have originally contemplated."[98] A little fancy, perhaps, but almost the very words of Sherlock Holmes. Concluding the interview, Dr. Bell mused, "You cannot expect the ordinary 'bobby,' splendid fellow as he is so far as pluck and honesty go, to stand eight hours on his legs, and then develop great mental strength, he doesn't get enough blood to his brain to permit of it." Again he agrees with Holmes about the positive character of the average policeman.

Like the great detective, Joe Bell "was much interested in the reading of character through handwriting and composition." He would send the myriads of letters that he received—with the senders' names erased—to Mrs.Saxby, who was also interested in the analysis of handwriting. She was impressed far more with what his friends were revealing about Bell than with his superb analyses.One patient wrote: "I take no credit to myself at all.... You start me afresh." Another wrote, "I thank you for making it possible for me to make up the past; I was drifting on and on, but you saved me. You so tempered justice with mercy. God bless you."

He, too, quite a few years before Mr. Holmes appeared in print, was tempering justice with mercy—later, of course, a Sherlock Holmes trademark.

Without realizing how much she was saying, Mrs.

Saxby once observed, "As amateur detective, he never brought the wrong-doer to public justice" [how wrong she was]; and "he tried to help the poor, the weak and the criminals brought before him. One of his favorite sayings was: 'We must not give the poor soul away'."[99] Here the good doctor sounds far more like Father Brown than Sherlock Holmes, but he often behaved more like the Prelate than the Detective. Dr. Bell also had a lukewarm belief in physiognomy, but not the extent of Mr. Holmes' reliance upon pugnacious jaws, determined chins, cauliflowered ears and thick lips. One of the most priceless lines in all of Sherlock Holmes is Dr. Mortimer's comment upon Mr. Holmes' own features when first those two worthies meet in *The Hound of the Baskervilles*: "You interest me very much, Mr. Holmes. I had hardly expected as dolicocepholic a skull.... A cast of your skull, Sir, until the original is available, would be an ornament to any anthropological museum." Both men, ironically enough, dealt with "wrong-doers" and "culprits," and both read the *Police News* with interest. Both were extremely impatient with bunglers, and felt one need tell a soul anything only *once*.

Like his friend and student Conan Doyle, Joseph Bell not only tried to concoct plots for detective stories,[100] he had a surprising knowledge of detective fiction. In the 1892 introduction Dr. Bell observed: "We may admire Lecoq, but we do not see ourselves in his shoes.... Voltaire taught us the method of *Zadig*[101] and every good teacher of medicine or surgery exemplifies every day in his teaching and practice the method and its results."

Also like Conan Doyle, he was a great admirer of Sir Walter Scott, advising Mrs. Saxby that "he [Scott] is a fine, wholesome, level-headed man, and I read his books not because they are stories, but because they are human."

Like Doyle, he was interested in homespun and

medieval romance: "But in the last few years," he says in
the introduction to the 1892 *Study in Scarlet*, "there has
been a distinct demand for books, which, to a certain poor
extent, encourage thought and stimulate observation.
The whole *Gamekeeper at Home* series[102] and its
imitations opened the eyes of town dwellers, who had
forgotten or never known White of Selborne,[103] to the
delightful sights and sounds that were the harvest of the
open eye and ear. Something of the same interest is given
to the 'crowded city's horrible street' by the suggestions of
crime and romance, of curiosity and its gratification,
which we find written with more or less cleverness in the
enormous mass of so-called detective literature under
which the press groans." (Doyle said practically the same
thing to his mother about Fergus Hume's runaway
detective best-seller *The Adventure of the Hansom Cab*.)
Conan Doyle, who wanted to be known for his historical
novels, appreciated this statement from Dr. Bell's
introduction the most: "If in addition the doctor is also a
born storyteller, then it is a mere matter of choice whether
he writes detective stories or keeps his strength for a great
historical romance as is the *White Company*." The author
replied to Bell's statement in the most celebrated letter he
wrote to Dr. Bell, the one of May 4, 1892, in which he tells
his former mentor he was the model for Sherlock Holmes.
He goes on to say: "I was so pleased too that you like *The
White Company* into which I put more heart and work
than into anything else I have done." On the other hand,
Doyle's ego also would have been puffed by the last
observation in the "Introduction": "The ordinary
detective story from Gaboriau or Boisgobey[104] down to the
latest shocker, really needs an effort of memory quite
misplaced to keep the circumstances of the crimes and the
wrong scents of the various meddlers before the wearied
reader. Dr. Doyle never gives you a chance to forget an
incident or miss a point." It would seem that all three

gentlemen were walking encyclopedias of the "great cases" and the great writers.

Throughout the early clamor his one big worry was that the reporters would start hounding his children. Fortunately the journalists were not all as intrepid as Mr. Harry How. Dr. Bell was busier than ever in his private practice, and spending more and more time at the Royal Hospital for Sick Children. Early in the new year he completed the two monographs that were requested by the medical profession of Edinburgh: "Five Years Surgery in the Royal Hospital for Sick Children" and the indispensible "The Surgical Side of the Royal Infirmary of Edinburgh, 1854-1892; the Progress of a Generation." (Like Mr. Holmes it seems he was a master of the monograph.) In April he delivered the valedictory address for the Medico-Chirurgical Society. On February 7, 1893 his older daughter Jean went through almost a carbon-copy of her sister's marriage, for then she too married a captain in The Royal Scots, Captain Harry McCance, in scenic Joslin Chapel at Milton Bridge.

In June of 1893, his son Benjamin, to whom the doctor was devoted, developed complications from an appendicitis attack, and died from peritonitis. In his Journal Joe Bell described the onset of his son's complications in his typical terse manner, but three of his colleagues (including Patrick Heron Watson) and Mrs. Saxby said, years later, they could not repeat the notes that Joe Bell sent them. All agreed that he aged appreciably. Robert Louis Stevenson, who evidently knew Joe Bell far better than we have been led to believe, wrote to an old Academy Friend on September 6, 1894 from Samoa:

Do you know I was greatly pleased with the little Academy paper? It was extremely interesting to see the old names repeated, some I was sure I could identify for certain, others I could only guess at. And there was one paragraffe [sic] which caused me a great deal of pain—I mean the death of Joe Bell's son. I wish you could find a way to communicate my sincere sympathy to Joe Bell. I doubt if I shall hear "The Flowers of the Forest" again without remembering him and his only son.[105]

The "Flowers of the Forest" was indeed played by two pipers of the 91st Highlanders, according to the *Edinburgh Academy Chronicle*, and "six sergeants of that regiment carried the coffin, covered with the Union Jack... and no more impressive scene could be imagined as the mourners passed slowly from the gate to the grave." While his son was christened Benjamin and seemed destined to become a physician, "if he ever regretted this break in the [medical] line he never spoke of it to anyone."[106] Again, his abiding faith sustained him, and he buried himself in his work.

He was fortunate that he chose such a course, for in August of 1893 he was called in as a forensics expert in "the biggest crime of the decade," the Monson case. It was a trial that had its rude beginning in 1890, when Major Dudley Hambrough, a wealthy London financier, hired a penniless young Oxford graduate named Alfred Monson to tutor his seventeen-year-old son, Cecil, for the Hampshire Militia. The scene shifted to Scotland three years later when the father leased Ardlamont House in Scotland in his son's name for a season of shooting.

In August of 1893, after having failed on two earlier attempts, Monson took out a £20,000 ($100,000) insurance police on the life of his pupil. He quite truthfully told the Glasgow manager of the New York Mutual Assurance Company that the boy stood to inherit $1,000,000 and that Mrs. Monson had advanced the boy significant sums in the past against that inheritance. Therefore, to protect the advance, the Monsons naturally wanted to insure the boy. The company bought the story, insured the pupil, and had the young man undergo two medical examinations. One wonders what Mr. Monson must have been telling young

Hambrough. Monson then paid the insurance company approximately £950 and the game was afoot.

A few days after paying the premium, Monson, a most capable swimmer, took his charge, a non-swimmer, on a fishing expedition—out in a rowboat. The boat suddenly sprang a leak, took on water and finally capsized. Fortunately for young Hambrough they were close to land and he was able to save himself by clinging to some rocks. The next morning, perhaps to make up for lost time, young Hambrough, his tutor, and a man named Scott (a mysterious, mustachioed engineer who disappeared for over a year) went shooting, although by all accounts the mysterious Mr. Scott carried no weapon. Monson carried a 12-bore shotgun, and his young pupil toted a 20-bore weapon. A few hours later Monson returned from the nearby woods and said in an even tone that young Hambrough was dead. At the trial Monson declared that he and his pupil had separated; he heard a shot; he ran in the direction of the blast: "I then saw Hambrough lying at the bottom of the sunk fence on his left side, with his gun beside him," Monson claimed. "We lifted him up, and he was quite dead."

Ironically it was accepted that the death of young Hambrough was accidental. Allowing a short time to expire, Monson filed a claim for the £20,000 insurance. He was informed that the deceased was a minor and thus the policy was invalid. One would think that Monson would have checked into the provisions of the policy with infinite care. In a trial that was replete with oddities, Monson said he was aware of the provisions, but wanted to try to bluff the company out of the money. It was at this point that the company became suspicious, and "a month later Sir Henry Littlejohn and Dr. Bell exhumed the body and re-examined the remains."[107] They took one look and agreed it was "murder most foul."

The Crown got out its big guns. They asked Sir Henry,

Dr. Bell, and one of the great ballistics experts of the day, Dr. Patrick Heron Watson, to testify. In the words of the *London Morning Leader's* sub-head: "They all [three doctors] agreed that Hambrough Could Not Have Accidentally Caused the Wounds, and that the Gun was Fired by an Assailant Who Stood Behind Him."[108]

First, Dr. Littlejohn took the stand, and described all the medical findings, and rendered his opinion that the shot came from too far away (at least eight feet) for Hambrough to have killed himself. He brought a skull into court with him to prove his point. "Dr. Patrick Heron Watson," the *Morning Leader* reported, "was next called. It is a strange coincidence that this friend of Dr. Bell, the original of Sherlock Holmes, is of the same name as Holmes's laborious and faithful chronicler. 'My dear Watson' is an expert in gunshot wounds." He too brought a skull with him into the courtroom. He, like Joe Bell and Dr. Littlejohn, pointed out that the triangular wound undoubtedly was made by stray pellets from a cartridge, many of which missed the skull of young Hambrough. "As was only appropriate," the *Morning Ledger* continued, "after Dr. Watson came Sherlock Holmes—Dr. Joseph Bell—a tall thin man, with narrow face, benevolent looking, with white hair, but with a preternaturally keen and eager look. He had a curious little trick of holding on to the front of the witness-box with his hands and swaying himself backwards and forward, coming forward in answer to a question and leaning back in the interval between one question and the next." The bulk of Joe Bell's testimony was a minute examination of the triangular wound. Taking great pains, he pointed out that because of the lack of powder burns on the skull, because only a part of the skull was shot away, that the shot would have come from at least ten feet away. Had Hambrough killed himself the shot would have come

from two or three feet away, and would have shattered his
skull. He discussed the thickness of the skull. Not unless
the young Mr. Hambrough had abnormally long arms
could he have shot himself. "The body of the shot," he
went on in his official testimony, "went right through the
bone *en balle*; having struck, four pellets appear to have
entered the aperture, and the rest to have gone into
space." The *Morning Leader* echoed the tension and
excitement of the proceedings: "The case was getting
grislier than ever, and the hand of Dr. Bell, the Sherlock
Holmes of the case—and the original of Dr. Conan Doyle's
creation—was plainly to be seen in the sequence with
which the investigations had been pursued." By the time
Joe Bell testified, the *Morning Leader* noted, "all the
doctors in the case have their particular skulls, which
they bring into the witness-box and put in their hats when
not in use. This makes the fourth skull in court besides
poor Hambrough's." Prominently featured in the
Morning Leader's account were pictures of Dr. Littlejohn
and Dr. Bell.

The Crown called in well over 100 witnesses, and tried
to demonstrate that after unsuccessfully trying to drown
poor Hambrough by boring a hole in the skiff and pulling
the plug, Monson did successfully shoot and kill the
young man and diabolically tried to palm it off as an
accident. If ever there seemed to be the proverbial open-
and-shut case this was it, but the presiding judge, Lord
Kinsburgh, was presiding over his first trial, and "in his
reminiscences, later, he admitted lying awake nights in
'dull perspiration, turning things over and over.' In his
final charge, preferring a safe and sure verdict, he
reminded the jury not to be swayed from justice by
Monson's bad character."[109] The jury deliberated about
eighty minutes, and came back with a "Not proven on
both charges"—a Scottish verdict, indicating lack of
sufficient evidence.

Wallace, who did an amazing amount of "on-location" investigation, is wrong when he says Dr. Bell told his wife that Monson got off because it was the judge's first case. Edith, of course, had died nearly twenty years earlier, but Drs. Bell, Littlejohn and Watson told all who would listen that they were convinced the judge was timorous because it was his first case. Mr. Wallace concludes his account of the trial by noting that Dr. Bell "was pleased to learn that Monson eventually wound up in prison for again attempting to defraud an insurance company." This time—absolutely true, but Dr. Littlejohn was far more elated. In fact, compared to the reactions of Sir Henry and Dr. Watson, Joe Bell was a stoic.

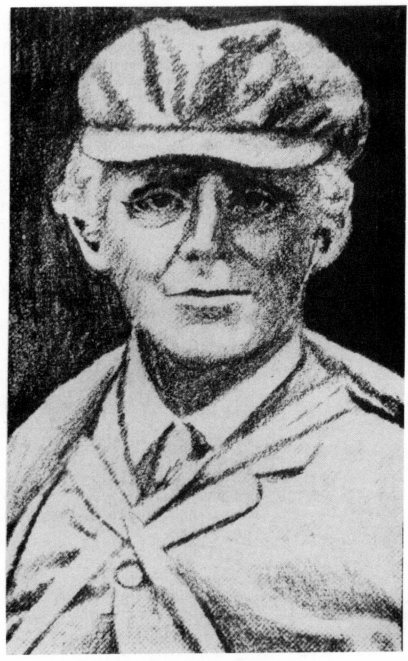

Joe Bell, grandfather, in his walking rig.

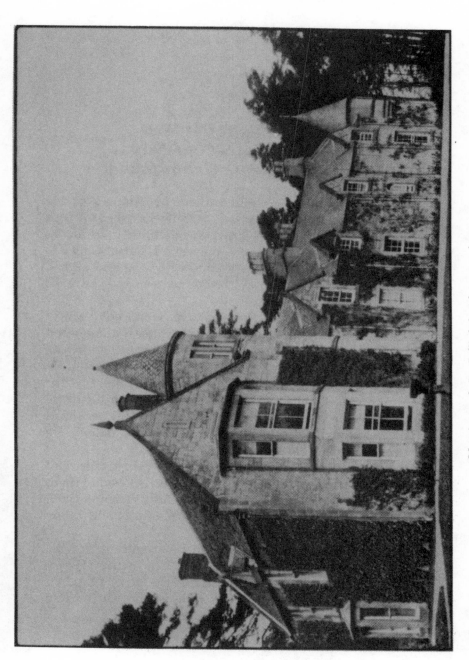

Mauricewood, Joe Bell's beloved summer home.

XI

The Valley Afar:
The Yellow-Leaf Days
of a Religious Grandfather

From veiled allusions and rather coy remarks to his colleagues and to Mrs. Saxby, Dr. Bell was asked to "look into" more cases for the Crown at this time.[110] Whatever they were, he seemed to enjoy the work. He also seemed to have more time to visit Jean and Cecil. Over and over in his later years, he wrote, "I hope to see Cecil & Co. in Kent."

The children looked forward to his visits, but it was at this time, 1894, that he decided to purchase Mauricewood outright, probably for the grounds and flowers as much as the gorgeous, multi-gabled house. In 1894 it would be called a country estate. One colleague, probably Dr. Annandale, said he moved to Mauricewood mainly to see how fast the horses could travel. Because of his penchant for carriages, his grandchildren called him "Gigs." He loved it.

These were probably the happiest days of his life, said his granddaughter Edith Fulton. "How he loved to romp here with his grandchildren; to welcome his friends. Such its delights, his garden might have been the island valley of Avilon."[111]

He counted among his friends, according to Mrs. Fulton, Robert Louis Stevenson, the witty Henry Littlejohn, Dr. Alexander Whyte, and the famous English actress Ellen Terry, and, so it would seem he was far from

being unhappy in his famed role as model for the great
Sherlock Holmes. Indeed, according to Mrs. Fulton, he
wanted very much to meet the celebrated American actor
who portrayed Holmes for nearly half a century—the
great William Gillette. It would also seem he maintained
his fine sense of humor, for the gardener's daughter at
Mauricewood, a Charlotte Brown, recalls that "on leaving
of a morning for Edinburgh, the doctor would pull up at
the gardener's lodge and call out [in his best Ward XI
manner]: 'Any orders today, Brown?' " From Mrs. Fulton
also we learn of his great love of animals, especially dogs,
and in the 1890s "he was to be seen every day seated in his
carriage on his way to Morningside Drive [site of the
Royal Hospital for Sick Children].... There was no
mistaking [his] conveyance even half way down the
Drive; it was invariably followed by a couple of Gordon
[sic] setters." On the grounds of Mauricewood today one
can see the plot set aside as the last resting place for
household pets. "The lairs," as the Evening News
observes, "are marked by stone slabs; 'Bones' is the not
inappropriate inscription on one; a second pays tribute to
a faithful friend and companion. Bishop by name."

In 1895 he was chosen by his fellowgraduates to be
one of the four University of Edinburgh assessors, a post
which he held till his death, and one that he said (quite
often) was the most important post of his life. In addition
to his counsel on University matters, his great medical
knowledge, tact and knowledge of the City made him a
"natural" for the University liaison man (there being no
women assessors). It seemed he knew everyone in the
City. One has to wonder at his stamina: forty-two years as
Examiner for The Royal College of Surgeons, Assessor on
the University Court for his last sixteen years, and yet,
says Sir William Turner, he "retained to the last his
quickness of apprehension, the power of expressing his
views with brevity and lucidity, and the geniality and

heartiness which characterized him throughout his long and useful life."

Truly putting his Christian faith in practise, he became well-known for taking care of the poor as well as the rich, treating all children and parents alike at the Royal Hospital for Sick Children, and, of course, his charitable work for the Royal Hospital for Incurables. His father had set him a good example. In later years, Dr. Caird said that when he spoke of Joe Bell's charity he thought of the poor that Dr. Bell would never charge. In his personal papers, Joe Bell had many scraps and snippets from patients who had kind words for him. One was a poem that makes a comment, and it drew a comment from Joe Bell:

Just yet compassionate, gentle yet firm and strong,
O'er coming ill by good, enduring long
Such grief must be, sent by Heaven's command,
Even as the Lancet in his skillful hand
Puts Death to flight; and if sore pain must be,
He courage lends by sweetest sympathy.

Blessings from Prince and Peasant are his share,
Equal their need, equal his loving care:
Long as life last shall grateful bosoms swell
Let one but whisper, 'Here is Dr. Bell.'

On the reverse side of the poem, he wrote (to a friend): "Written by a somewhat daft old Lady whose family I have looked after for nothing for years."

He too turned more and more to his own poetry when he "rode out to Mauricewood." It was still somewhat sentimental, with definite religious overtones (or undertones), but it is reassuring to know that doctors do such things. In 1895 he penned the following:

Give me, dear Lord, thy magic common things
Which all can see, which all may share;

Sunlight and dewdrops, grass and stars and sea,
Nothing unique or new, and nothing rare.

Just daisies, Knapweed, wind among the thorns,
Some clouds to cross the blue old sky above;
Rain, winter fires, a useful hand, a heart,
The common glory of a woman's love.

Then, when my feet no longer tread new paths
(Keep them from fouling sweet things anywhere)
Write one old epitaph in grace-lit words:
"Such things look fairer that he sojourned here."

Since in many ways, Joe Bell sounds almost too good
to be true or a man without a blemish, it would be well to
examine as many sides as possible, especially from a man
who was naturally shy, modest and unassuming. In the
1890s he corresponded more with Mrs. Saxby, and more
observations turn up by friends and colleagues. For some
reason he comments far more frequently about world
events. To the modern reader many of the views
contradict what he or correspondents said about his
"world outlook." At times he sounds naive, but that's from
a twentieth-century point of view. "Poor Dreyfus," he
writes to Mrs. Saxby in the late 90s. "It is a terrible tale,
and yet France is not all base and cruel. Their army
generals seem to be a rotten crew at present, and need to be
taught a lesson. No doubt you are right that there is much
of the tiger nature in a Frenchman, but even Tigers have
good traits."

He seems to have gotten quite excited over the Russo-
Japanese War, and followed it as closely as he did the U.S.
Civil War. He just had more to say about it: "As for the
newspaper, many of them are below contempt in their
partisanship, and especially in their putting in their
columns such a variety of obvious lies. They seem to
expect us to believe anything the cunning Asiatic likes to
tell.... I am so sorry for the Tzar. He is between the devil

and the deep sea—Socialists and his army. I am sure they [the Russian fleet] don't hanker after a fight with Admiral Togo.... I fear the old story, 'Nicky [the Tzar] ran away' is still true."[112]

On the subject of the Boer War, Dr. Bell sounds like an echo of his prize pupil, Conan Doyle. Doyle, of course, was knighted for his astounding work in setting up a field hospital in South Africa and for his many books and pamphlets justifying England's role in the War. The war, according to both men, would have been over sooner but for "traitors" at home. Both, however, in Dr. Bell's words, felt "for the Boers, they have fought fairly and gallantly. It won't be a pleasure trip to Praetoria as some thought but it is bound to come off in time." Then, getting truly worked up, he continues, "You surely don't want us to be kicked out of South Africa. Once a nation begins to give in, it is a dying nation, and soon will be a dead one.... Would you have approved of Kruger[113] invading Natal 'to eat fish at Durban'—as the Boers said they meant to do? The end is in sight, don't fear, and the natives will get a chance of decent treatment...."[114]

At times he seems quite surprised to find others praising his long-time friend Mrs. Saxby—as a naturalist, a solid critic, and as a reformer. (In 1932, when she was over 90, Mrs. Saxby's hometown of Unst in the Shetland Islands celebrated her literary achievements—over 200 books, articles, essays. The headlines in the *Shetland Times* for Saturday, September 24 screamed: "Happy Function at Wullver's Hool"—Mrs. Saxby's home.) "I have read your last letter in the *Scotsman* about the school bairns. You make out a good case. I wish all weans could have dry boots and a good luncheon.... I read your letters in the *Scotsman,* and am astonished at the variety and accuracy of your knowledge. Tom Speedy vouches for you as a naturalist, and he knows." His taste in writers, if a small sampling is typical, ran a little more to the religious and historical than "intellectual." He again wrote Mrs. Saxby, "You have made good use of the library, and the criticisms are capital, especially on poor J.S. Mill's biography. It is a very sad book, and he wasn't what one might call a 'wise body.' When clever men go off the beaten track they often get lost in a marsh.... The three books (new ones) I have liked most this year have been 'Theophrastus Such,' 'Dean Hook's Life' and S. Wilberforce's 1st vol.... It is most fascinating, and he must have been a 'real nice' man, though with his weaknesses."[115]

Much has been said of Joe Bell's religion, his charitableness, and his compassion. Nathan Bengis, one of the most indefatigable Sherlockian scholars, said in a review (a rather late review) of Mrs. Saxby's book that Joe Bell could not tolerate formalism. Mrs. Saxby repeatedly said Dr. Bell was broad-minded, and so it is curious that no one has commented on his reply to her questionaire-game when she threw out to him: "Nation Most Disliked." His answer: "Polish Jews and Connaught Irish." Quite a combination. Without trying to get the good doctor off any kind of hook, Joe Bell was not the most liberal of churchmen and did not pretend to be. While he said little about the Irish, he did comment on the Jews a few times. Writing to Mrs. Saxby upon receipt of the manuscript of her latest novel in 1892, *Heim-Laund* and *Heim Folk*, he said:

Your manuscript arrived safely.... I can't recall any such incidents in my reading; but I don't know Jewish history well except from the Bible.... You know your ground.

Many thanks for telling me the sources of your Jew novel. Your imagination is most vivid, and I am sure you are right in your conclusions.... I, like you, are a great believer in the Jews. They have kept up their race so splendidly, and are always looking still for the Messiah. Yes, they do indeed inherit the Promises, and someday these will be fulfilled, as you say, to astonish the Gentiles.

He had seen few, if any, Polish Jews. The Jews started leaving Russia and Poland in the '80s (mainly because of intense government persecution) for the United States, and some wound up in Scotland, mostly in Glasgow. The sight of a man with his black caftan, the long black robe; the wide-brimmed fur hat; and flowing earlocks would have been as alien to Joe Bell as seeing a man from Mars. Hearing them would have been even stranger, for their Scots-Yiddish dialect would defy the best of linguists. The great literary scholar David Daiches, whose father was Chief Rabbi in Edinburgh, gives us a fine example of an argot that would have left the good doctor scratching his head: "Aye mon; ich habe getrebbled mit de 5 o'clock train [I took/traveled on the 5 o'clock train]; and "Ye'll hae a drop of bramfen [whisky], eh? Nem a schmeck [take a taste]. It's Dzon Beck [John Begg], ye ken."[116]

Daiches recorded the most significant statement at the beginning of his delightful article: "Edinburgh, one of the few European capitals with no tradition of anti-semitism, accepted them [Jewish immigrants] with a characteristic cool interest."[117]

Mr. Bengis' comment about Dr. Bell's not being able to tolerate formalism is a fortuitous opening to the whole subject of Dr. Bell's religion. Just as Conan Doyle left the Catholic faith for his own brand of religion and later Spiritualism (he had an abhorrence of atheists), Joe Bell's father left the Calvinistic tenets of the official Scottish Church for the Free Church.[118] Both breaks were hard ones; they changed the courses of lives radically.

Joe Bell was born into the Free Church faith. He was "ever interested in the Bible" according to his father; shone in Biblical Studies at the Academy; and was quick to quote the Bible upon every occasion.[119] He had an unshakeable faith in the World to Come, but had Parson Adams' firm belief that man's grace shone ever more brightly when he helped his fellow man. Good deeds were essential. Often he was in charge of his siblings in church, and there was absolutely no need for Benjamin Bell to tell the children to behave there. Decorum reigned. While it may have been the norm, or at least not unusual, to attend services twice on Sundays at St. George's Free Church, it will probably surprise the modern churchgoer to learn that "it was normal to queue up to get into St. George's West for the evening Service."[120]

St. George's West, "quite a famous preaching station," was located at the western end of Edinburgh's famed Princes Street, just off Lothian Road. In the pulpit for most of Joe Bell's adult years was the equally famed and exciting minister Alexander Whyte, who had succeeded the eloquent Reverend Candlish in 1869. Dr. Bell's granddaughter, Mrs. Fulton, remembers her grandfather arguing for "hours on end" with Dr. Whyte. While she did not know the nature of the arguments, she knew whatever it was was important and significant in the lives of each. They were debating the very essence of their religion: grace, the Trinity, salvation, the role of the minister, etc. No subject was closer to Joe Bell's soul. For a relatively calm man, this was one subject that could destroy his inner peace.

Dr. Alexander Whyte, *sans peur* and *sans reproche*, had one of the strangest backgrounds in Edinburgh, a city that looked askance at any blot on any scutcheon. Dr. Bell knew quite well a bit about Dr. Whyte's antecedents, for he was a man whom people trusted. He was a good listener, and one of the strangest stories he ever heard came from Dr. Whyte's lips during the early days of their friendship. The two met in Glasgow, and like so many others, Dr. Whyte began confiding in Joe Bell almost from the day they met. It was the American Civil War that first drew them together.

Joe Bell learned that John Whyte, the minister's father, left Scotland before the boy was born. He had never married Dr. Whyte's mother (it was more or less a question of pride on at least one side), but instead ran off to America—to Pennsylvania, New Jersey, New York. At the start of the Civil War John Whyte enlisted, becoming "the Comasary of the 79th Regiment, Highland Guard, New York State Militia," and sporting a full beard, a black service cap, and, fittingly enough, "a kilt and a colossal sporran hanging far below his knees," he went off to war.[121] He was decorated for bravery, eventually captured and imprisoned by the Confederates in two thoroughly unsanitary prisons. Later Dr. Bell and all of Dr. Whyte's intimate friends were overjoyed to learn of Dr. Whyte's reunion with his father (albeit brief). The elder Whyte was then suffering from a bone disease brought on by his confinement in the Confederate prisons. The Reverend Whyte also met his half-sister, who came over from America.[122]

Ever a friend to the Reverend, Joe Bell was never too busy or shy, as we have seen from Mrs. Fulton, to argue his conscience with Dr. Whyte. Dr. Whyte, to his credit, was a fierce champion of absolute freedom of the pulpit. In the summer and fall of 1887, however, when his professional life was changing so dramatically, Joe Bell "really got into it," with Dr. Whyte at a time when he, Joe Bell, badly needed a complete rest. Dr. Alexander Whyte had met with a fiery Irishman by the name of John Dillon. Dillon was organizing a "Plan of Campaign" by which thousands of crofters [renters of small, enclosed farms] were to join in a rent strike to enforce attention to their demands for the abolition of rent-racking [rents equal to the value of nearly all the land] on the part of their British landlords. Mr. Dillon "expressed his wonder not less than his gratification, that he should thus find himself a welcome guest of such a gathering in a Scottish Presbyterian Manse."[123]

Although the meeting (with several leading

ministers) was strictly private, at least thirteen members
of St. Georges, including eight Elders, drew up a long
"remonstrance" against the behavior of their minister.
Joe Bell was one of them.

They felt Mr. Dillon's opinions and projects "not
merely unpatriotic and dangerous from a political point of
view, but as contravening fundamental laws of public and
private morals."[124] They were, however, essentially
concerned with the graver problem of how far a
clergyman ought to give active support to a political party
or movement in matters of acute public controversy.

They began their remonstrance by flatly asserting
that he couldn't get involved without compromising the
congregation, and observing that he had been hired for
graver concerns than secular politics, but they conclude
with the temporizing observation: "No one would ever
think of questioning your sacred right of individual
opinion and of supporting that opinion by your vote, but
we venture to submit to you that many considerations ...
point to the high expediency of our minister abstaining
himself in so marked a manner as you have recently done
with *either side* of any burning political controversy."

While Dr. Whyte went on to defend Robertson Smith,
a minister whose critical views and emendations of the
Bible shocked many a Scottish layman (especially the
issue of a non-Mosaic authorship of *Deuteronomy*), he
kept a low profile, as it were, on all political issues
thereafter. He was, however, always forthright, with little
patience for the "somewhat timid proprieties of Victorian
Edinburgh." He attacked vice and corruption in the city,
calling a spade a spade. Even college students felt he
wielded the prophet's scourge too openly, and admitted
many young people were shaken to the foundations of
their being "by some of Dr. Whyte's addresses on personal
morality." Even when addressing a group of men only he
used a language starkly frank, and direct, and rare for

that time. One of the most effective of his soul-searching questions: "Young man, what will you think of this on your wedding morning?"

He could shake the rafters on allied subjects at St. George's too, and we find Dr. Benjamin Bell, an Elder before his son, writing thus to his minister: "I cannot help telling you how much I appreciated your discourse... on the seventh commandment. It was *masterly*, and I know it must have been the outcome of much prayer and consideration.... I write this, notwithstanding your warning ... against flattery, to let you know what one, who does not stand alone, thought of it."[125] One Dissenter called Dr. Whyte "The *non plus ultra* of Dissenters: a Dissenter among Disrupters." It may be well here, since St. George's was quarreling with part of the Scottish or Presbyterian Church, to elucidate what "The Disruption," as the Free Church Revolt (1843) was called, really meant. The rebels who formed the Free Church in 1843 "were men of absolute conviction and courageous temper.... The principle on which they stood was that 'no minister shall be intruded into any parish contrary to the will of the congregation'... the principle of democracy, that is—and when the government of their day refused their claim to spiritual independence, 470 ministers walked out, with no promise of [making a living]... other than the goodwill of equally independent worshippers, and proceeded to build new churches and establish a new and somewhat narrow rule."

Joe Bell loved to recall the sing-song name-calling or badinage that took place when the new, Free Churches were erected—having small pretensions, as one historian says, to architectural dignity: "The Free Kirk, the wee kirk, the kirk wi'oot a steeple," chanted the establishment regulars. "The Auld Kirk, the cauld kirk, the kirk wi'oot the people," retorted the rebels, and the fight was on.[126] He felt the Established Church was "making great strides" and was quite "as evangelical as our U.F." He thought they would eventually merge. On this point, Mrs. Saxby after averring that Joe Bell was indeed loyal to his church, "but broadminded to a degree," goes on to point out a different line of his religious thought:

> About the divisions in the Church he once wrote: 'These divisions of Churches seem to me most futile and trifling, but terribly bad for religion.... Of course, you agree with me that the split in our Kirks is giving the game to the enemy.
> If one could only swallow the Roman Catholic 'whole' how sweet it would be! But one can't put one's conscience in the hands of a priest. And a Pope! No! All that posturing, and dressing up, and ancient fables—a sane mind can't accept all that.... A person of your sort must avoid the fascination of Rome. They are a clever lot, those priests, and I don't say they are wrong. Some I know are Saints on earth, and shame our ministers often with their self-sacrifycing lives. But they want converts.... How would you like to be in Purgatory for any indefinite number of years? If your friends neglected to pay for your Masses, *there* you might stick.'

From the accounts of others, he became more and more impressed with the efforts of the priests for the poor and their warm relationship with their flock. He seems never to have attended a Mass, but instead became ever more active in his own Church, and even on his two-week honeymoon throughout Scotland, he recorded his hearing "Mr. Greig preach twice" and, seven days later, "Twice at Church. Mr. Trail [spoke] on James 1:22." Let it be said that on that same honeymoon he called on Dr. Lister and Dr. Gairdner when he and Edith were in Glasgow.

Much has been made of his charity and compassion. He evidently had worked out a typical Joe Bell kind of program on charity. He and Edith, as pointed out, had vowed to give a tenth of their income "for God's service." He contributed to at least three hospitals and gave of his free time to two of them. He evidently "gave in secret," feeling that was the way of true charity. Charity, of an even higher nature he felt, like Shaw and Maimonides, was helping people help themselves: helping the poor get jobs. "His generosity," wrote a colleague, "no one can measure. It was all done so unostentatiously, so tactfully, that none but the recipient knew of it." Dr. Kellman, a minister from New York, of all places, who succeeded Alexander Whyte, also said that "his generosity was as lavish as it was secret." It is interesting that the will he made out in 1896 was altered in 1902 and 1909. Originally he left Janet Campbell, "my faithful servant," £20 a year and Matthew Burton, his butler, £100. All the other servants were to receive a year's wages at his death. By 1909 the faithful servants' largess was doubled, and Matthew Burton was to receive £250. In 1909, a gardener at Mauricewood, Thomas Davie, was left a considerable sum; and James Inglis, a coachman, was bequeathed £100. George Pack, now writing a history of Egerton, recalls another instance of Dr. Bell's generosity:

> Dr. Bell, remember, was frequently a visitor to Egerton House [home of Cecil and her husband, Major Stisted]: My father, who was a groom at the time, would be sent in company with the coachman and a carriage and a pair of horses to Lenham Station to pick the Dr. up from the train. At the end of his visit, before being taken back to catch his train, the parlour maid would be sent to the stables with the instructions that Dr. Bell wished to see my father at the front door (it was always the front door). Upon meeting him there, the Dr. would give my father a half sovereign. At the time my father's wage was two shillings and sixpence per week... so this gift was a month's wages.

Evidently his "bedside manner" was also one of compassion. Patients praised his kind hands, his kind words. Jessie Saxby's husband, also a physician, became very ill a little after the Saxbys had just met Dr. Bell. The doctor and Mrs. Saxby realized her husband had a terminal illness. He advised her to be forthright and tell Mr. Saxby the nature of his illness. She could not do it.

" 'Very well, all right,' Joe Bell answered with a careless toss of his head. 'If *you* won't I must. It's in my line. All in the doctor's day's work, you know,' and he smiled.

"I thought, 'How callous.'

"Presently he said, 'Well, I must get to work. Let's go see him.' But when we reached the bedroom door he laid his hand on my shoulder, and said, 'Sit where I can't see your face when I am talking to him.'

"Behind the curtain I listened and marvelled at the tact, the gentleness, the knowledge of his patient's character, the hopefulness displayed. The bitter truth was suggested so calmly and carefully that before long my husband himself remarked most composedly, 'I suppose it is something of that sort that has me'."

Later Dr. Bell told Mrs. Saxby, "You were a brave child, and didn't make a fuss, and I did not see your face; but I saw your hands, and they said more than I like to think of."

Mrs. Saxby, a native of the Shetland Islands, knew that Joe Bell had spent some "pleasant holidays" at the Lunna estate in the Shetland Islands. Somehow he seemed to be able to reach the taciturn Islanders. They confided in him. "He was a busy, 'fame-encircled' doctor, but he gave—and more often than not for no remuneration—his time and careful attention to the folk who came from Shetland.... The gift of a pair of socks or gloves from a grateful patient evoked a warm acknowledgement out of all proportion to the poor woman's gift. 'Isn't this touching? I am delighted, and I hope the child will recover.... It was little I could do for it, but it refreshes me to find they like what I do'."

Many patients and friends were also attracted to another side of Joe Bell that bordered on Mysticism, a trait observed at least once by most of those who knew him. He was a soother, a calmer, one who inspired hope and confidence. Often he brought to bear several of his amazing talents to sooth the distraught friend or patient.

Once an Irish student came to him, upset that his girlfriend, whose letters had once been so affectionate, had just sent him a note, saying the two were not meant for each other. The poor boy could not put his mind to his studies or to anything. Dr. Bell asked to see the letter. He examined it carefully, and then told the lad not to worry. "Pay no attention to the letter," said the doctor, "for she still loves you very much." The young man was incredulous, but Joe Bell's skill at hand-writing analysis enabled him to conclude, from the wavering hand and the hectic punctuation, that the letter certainly had not been spontaneous. Indeed, the substance revealed, psychologically, that it may have been written under pressure. Learning more about the home situation, Dr. Bell told the astonished lad that the letter was dictated by the girl's mother, and that the young man be circumspect but not disheartened. He kept in touch with the girl, and was delighted to learn that the letter had indeed been dictated by an over-protective mother.[127]

Dr. Z.M. Hamilton, the Edinburgh-trained doctor, Sherlockian and Canadian historian, recalls the story of a young Scotsman named Campbell, who was disinherited by his mother who had remarried. The young man, then a student at the University, decided to go to Alberta, Canada after graduation because a friend had found him a position on the staff of a hospital there. The only thing standing between young Campbell and the job was an oral examination. Since the young man had a slight speech impediment that grew worse under stress, it was rather a formidable hurdle for him. The friend, Dr. Hamilton's aunt, wakened in the middle of the night and asked him to take a message to Dr. Joe Bell at Mauricewood. He got to the doctor's home in the middle of the night, and was surprised to hear the doctor order his carriage and pair. The two returned to Edinburgh immediately. The doctor insisted on hearing the aunt's analysis of the young man's problems and then young Campbell's version. The next day, showing no favor at all as one of the young man's examiners, he made young Campbell feel at ease and even confident. He passed his oral examination "with credit."

One of the most mystic stories concerns a parlour maid at Egerton House in Kent. The gardener, George Pack's father, recalls the maid was called away while doing some needlework. She returned and sat down in the chair where she had previously placed the needle. She immediately cried out in pain and jumped up. A search was made by some of the other servants to try to locate and remove the needle, but no sign of the needle could be found. Dr. Bell was just arriving at his daughter's home and was immediately summoned. He heard the entire story, talked to the maid, then "he just put his hands on the girl's shoulders and said, 'Don't worry, my girl, it will be quite all right now.' With this assurance the girl completely forget the incident, after staring deeply into the understanding eyes of the doctor.

Strictly on the basis of evidence in Mrs. Saxby's book, Nathan Bengis saw another "mystical" side to Dr. Bell: Spiritualism, or, as Mrs. Saxby styled it: Second Sight. It seems that ever since she was a child she had "the Powers" or Second Sight, and Dr. Bell was skeptical about it for a long time. He finally asked her to experiment, "and when I did so successfully, he willingly allowed there was something to it." If one reads carefully, however, Joe Bell really doesn't want to hurt his friend's feeling, for when a Professor Henry Sidgwick wished her to "perform" before the Psychical Society in Cambridge, he "put his foot down." It is hard to know if he didn't want to see her embarrassed or if he thought the Cambridge people were charlatans—probably the latter. "How do you know but that the deil's in it? And until you are sure he *isn't* in it, you should not tempt Providence. I allow it may be a scientific fact, as you persist in thinking, but science hasn't got a grip on it yet." Nowhere else does he ever talk about spiritualism, but when he tells his friends, "These psychical experts will play the mischief with you" and when he says, "Besides, I rather do think the deil *may* have a little to do with it," he sounds far removed from that True Believer of Spiritualism, A. Conan Doyle, who had given up on formal religion and would have no truck with "deils."

Later Mrs. Saxby tells us that Joe Bell wrote her and said, "Mind I am a real believer in it [White Magic, as he called it] now.... You ought to know that no wise man accepts a new theory without searching and exhaustive examination." Mrs. Saxby, however, had the good sense to see he might be humoring her on the subject: "Nevertheless, there was a good deal of quiet fun in the way he wrote of this mysterious power of mine... and he often qualified his approval by saying: 'I must see the science of it before I can be quite convinced'."

On the other hand, so changed has the world become, that few Christians would believe that some of his rock-firm religious tenets didn't smack of Spiritualism. He believed that the soul passes through no sudden or great change when it leaves the body, but "simply continues the life he led on earth in a pure atmosphere beyond the reach of all temptations, and that enables it progress in all manner of spiritual goodness" and as Mrs. Saxby says about his thoughts of Edith, "Her memory was cherished to the latest hour of his life, and he looked forward to their reunion as a literal fact about which there could be no doubt." He didn't feel one should say a lot about religion, as that other great topic on which to be silent—politics.

While he made it a point "never to talk politics," he was a well-known conservative, and succeeded his friend and colleague Dr. Annandale as Chairman of the University Conservative Association. His last act as

Chairman of that Association was to nominate his old friend Sir Robert Finlay, also an M.D. of Edinburgh, to represent the Parliamentary constituency of the University. It may not be totally erroneous to point out that while he was certainly not a party or even active politician, the *Times* in its obituary labelled him an Imperialist as well as a conservative. It was Jessie Saxby's view that he was liberal-minded as well as conservative, "ready to acknowledge the wisdom and justice of some Radical measures. He once wrote, 'And so you dare confess yourself a rabid Leebral. Well, there are saints as well as sinners among that crew. Some of my very good friends are on your side of politics. If you keep your mind open, and allow that we have something decent to say for ourselves, I shall not scold you."

XII

"Stand With Me Here on the Terrace": The Open Road, Open Graves, Old Memories

In 1896 Dr. Bell was not yet sixty, but he had been doing the work of three men. He begins speaking of being overworked and seeking rest: "About giving up work, I often think of it and would like a winter abroad; but I put it from me.... Moderate work seems the best for us on the whole." He resigned as editor of the *Edinburgh Medical Journal*, and then, as alluded to earlier, he was called in as "the Veritable Peacemaker" when troubles arose over reorganization and editorial policy. As the *Times* said of him: "Dr. Bell had unusual business capacity combined with good judgment and acumen, which led to his being constantly consulted by his professional brethren and others whenever an unusual difficulty arose." It was a year in which another edition of one of his books came out and was reviewed most favorably: the fourth edition of his *Nurses Manual*.

He had already been thinking of resigning from his position as Chief Surgeon of the Royal Hospital for Sick Children, and seemed to start winding down the clock when he did so early the next year. "Every child in Edinburgh is indebted to this great man," wrote his colleague and "friendly rival," Dr. John Chiene—"rich, poor, churched and unchurched." He became Consulting Surgeon to the rapidly growing institution, a position he held for the rest of his life. It should not be forgotten that

he had one of the largest private practices in Edinburgh at
this time—a time in which Joe Bell often made over
twenty house calls a day. He also began spending more
time in his chemical laboratory. Even on policy matters or
working conditions of the nurses he was still being
consulted. On January 13, 1897 Florence Nightingale
wrote him, expressing deep regret that his term of office
was over and hoped that no harm would befall Miss
Spencer, Matron. He assured her that nothing "in the
least bad" would happen to the Matron. Also before he
left, the King of Siam, after conferring with the Queen,
made sure he visited Joe Bell's surgical wards at the Royal
Hospital. His secretary, Frederick Verney, wrote to Dr.
Bell, informing him that "His Majesty the King of Siam
was very much interested in all that he saw yesterday at
the Children's Hospital, and desires me to convey his
thanks to yourself for the clear explanations you were
good enough to give when he went round the wards."

During the next ten years (which saw the new century
ushered in), he himself sadly noted he was writing more
and more to friends and relatives about the death of loved
ones, colleagues, former students. In 1899 he wrote,
"Thanks for your kind and loving sympathy which I
knew were mine. I was prepared for the loss, as months
ago I gave up hope. It is the first break in our family of
nine (aging 61-44), which is a remarkable record." This
was the death of his sister Maria Isabella, of whom he
said in his Journal: "Very clever. Never married." He was
also glad to see the "births," as it were: When the fifth
edition of the *Nurses Manual* came out in 1899, he gave
the usual "Laus Deo," and thought two new editions in
two years "most satisfying." It was about this time, too,
that the world, while waiting for more Sherlock Holmes,
continued reading about him. At the turn of the century
the good doctor was besieged by energetic, persistent
reporters, eager to learn more about the model. When the

Hound of the Baskervilles came out in 1902, Joe Bell found himself hounded too. The reading public couldn't get enough of the canny detective and anything or anyone connected with him.

Two years earlier, however, the mentor went to the aid of his former pupil in the political arena—not so much as a publicity ploy or as a measure of support, but as an outraged man of conscience. Conan Doyle was running (or "Standing," as the British would have it) for Parliament for the Liberal Unionist party from the Central Division of Edinburgh. Joe Bell did not become involved until a low blow was struck by a religious fanatic (not Doyle's opponent), according to John Dickson Carr.[128] Shortly before the election, posters were plastered all over Edinburgh, letting it be known that Mr. Doyle, after all, was a Papist. He was, in the language of one of the craftily conceived posters, "One of them Catholic fellers." He was also labeled (derisively): "Mr. Sherlock Holmes." He felt that his old student was attacked in the foulest manner possible. He detested bigots. "I have no patience with bigots," he wrote a friend. "There is some hypocrisy in conjunction with bigotry." So the good doctor stood beside the sturdy author on the steps of the Edinburgh Literary Institute on the night of October 1, 1900, and urged the audience to vote for Doyle, "my former dresser." He assured the audience, according to the *Scotsman*, that "if Conan Doyle does half as well in Parliament as he did in the Royal Edinburgh Infirmary, he will make an unforgettable impression on English politics (cheers)." Doyle, who had good reason to believe he was a sure winner before the smear campaign, lost to the Radical candidate, G.M. Brown, a publisher, by a 3,028 to 2,459 margin.

In 1902 Bell was besieged to write about his former student or do introductions to the many collections being published. When he found the time to relax he began doing that which many a person says he will do "some day." He began reading more of those he admired: Browning, Shakespeare, Scott and the Bible. He offered to read articles by his aspiring medical colleagues, and began correcting proof for his friend Mrs. Saxby, who by 1902 had turned out many volumes of fiction. He obviously had a fine literary instinct, according to the novelist, and didn't hesitate to write "gush" or "high falutin'" beside certain passages of her work. He was also the first to congratulate her on each new work: "I am so pleased with the splendid notices of the ... little book, and quite proud of the reflected glory on my humble effort at the end" (a poem he had written as a young man).

His armchair involvement in the Boer War and the Russo Japanese conflict seems to bear out Irving Wallace's notion that he was becoming a "crusty old widower" at this time, but only to a degree. He became a nore ardent, active tennis player, observing to a colleague, however, that it didn't take any time at all for him to become tired of any form of vigorous exercise.

About this time also Mrs. Saxby gave him the famous questionnaire-game. Some of his answers do bring out the pixy in the man:

Favorite Virtue...................... Loving-Kindness
Vice Most Disliked .... Hypocrisy.
Special Aversion .... Company Manners.
Special Weakness ...... Grouse shooting in September.
Favourite Hour.................... Between the Lights.
Ideal of Enjoyment...... What passeth understanding.
Ideal of Misery .... Self-consciousness.
The Life you Prefer..... A busy one with a spring in it.
Favourite Employment ...Consultations in the country.
Highest Worldly Aspiration . To keep out of the Calton Jail!

Your besetting sin ... Stinginess and general meanness.
Place you Like Best ...... Over the hills and far away.
What most excites your enthusiasm Facing fearful odds.
What most excites your pity? A modest student who yet
must be "plucked" [flunked.]

Early in July of 1904, he wrote: "Another sister gone.
She was very near to us all." This was Dora Cecelia, his
oldest sister. He later commented to a colleague how
strong some women can be at such times. He was
impressed by and grateful for his sole remaining sister's
help. This was Elizabeth Grace, ever referred to as Libby,
and of whom Joe Bell once wrote: "Very strong and
capable. Kept house for Laurence and Harry. Never
married." We have no idea how he felt about the return of
Sherlock Holmes from the dead (or at least the
Reichenbach Falls), except John Chiene's view that it was
a "Well, look who's back" reaction.

Like Conan Doyle, the doctor liked traveling and he
liked speed. As late as April, 1907 he was proudly posing
for pictures in his barouche and pair. Four months later,
in August, 1907, he bought an automobile, one of the first
in Edinburgh, and drove 30 miles. Thereafter his Journal
is full of references to the car. He hired a chauffeur,
Collingwood, and spent more time as a consultant in the
country and also spent more time visiting the Edinburgh
Hospital for Incurables. As late as September 10, 1911—
less than a month before his death—he wrote to a friend of
the joys of his garden at Mauricewood and the pleasure of
long motor drives in the glorious summer days. On
December 1, 1897, a day before his birthday, his brother
Laurie died. "It was a sad birthday as my sailor brother
died." Laurence (Laurie) Bell seemed to occupy a special
place in Joe Bell's heart. He joined the Royal Navy while a
very young man, and is referred to by Joe Bell in his will of

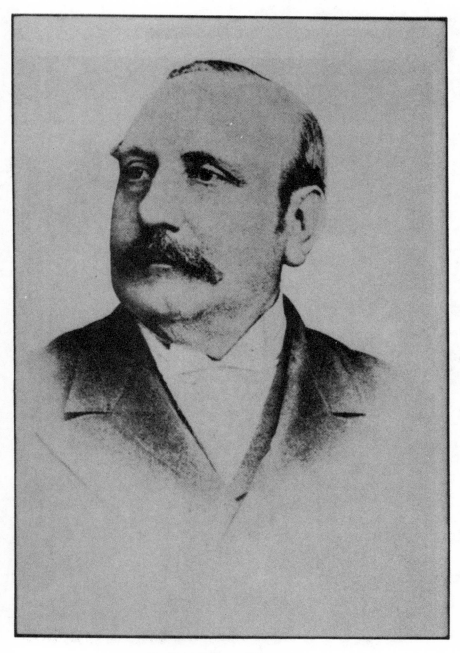

Dr. Patrick Heron Watson
"Fastest Knife in the West"

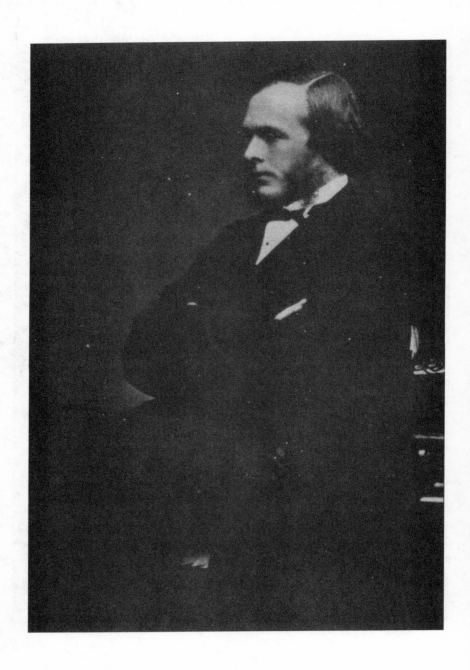

Baron Joseph Lister

1896 as "Retired Commander Royal Navy." Shortly thereafter, again with heavy heart, he wrote: "Then my old friends, Annandale and Heron Watson, died on successive days, and they were also buried in the Dean last Monday and Tuesday. So it has been a time of open graves and many old memories."

Patrick Heron Watson probably deserves a book unto himself, but certainly his connection with Joseph Bell and Arthur Conan Doyle deserves some space here. He was five years Joe Bell's senior, and at the Royal Infirmary he was known as Spence's boy, just as Dr. Bell was known as Syme's boy. Oddly enough, Spence was probably the Napoleon of surgeons in his generation, as Heron Watson was the greatest wielder of the scalpel in his. In this regard Joe Bell was truly the second most dexterous knife in Edinburgh. Watson, who had vied with the great Lister for the position of assistant surgeon and lost, succeeded Lister to that position when Lister was wooed away to Glasgow in 1860. Joe Bell, of course, later became Watson's assistant. Both men unsuccessfully applied for Syme's clinical Surgery Chair when that worthy died in 1869, and it was Lister again who got the position. Heron Watson was trained in preanesthetic conditions in the Crimea, and there he developed an operating technique that was probably the fastest of the century. "Spence," says Dr. C.E. Douglas, "could disarticulate the hip in six seconds, and Watson's hand was just as quick.[129] Memory recalls an amputation at the shoulder by Dr. Watson. There was a flash of the blade as it transfixed the deltoid: one's notebook dropped to the floor was hastily picked up, and in those seconds behold the arm, completely severed.... Another case comes back to memory," he continues: "A man is brought anesthetized into the theatre on a mattress. [Dr. Watson] strolls in, one hand in his pocket, stoops and examines the hip, gives a short description of a dislocation. He then takes the foot, sweeps the limb round in a wide circle, flexes the knee, and with another circular movement the head slips into place with consummate ease. Nothing ever disturbed a certain massive calm."

The "certain massive calm" could be seen in one of the favorite anecdotes ever at the Royal Infirmary. A patient was wheeled before Heron Watson for lithotomy. He was trussed up, and "Watson sits down," says Dr. Douglas, "and passes a finger into the rectum. The preliminary enema had not, it would seem, sufficiently cleared the rectum, and an unexpected deluge greets him. Consternation and breathless silence, as nurses rush to the rescue. Watson washes his hands, turns to the unfortunate resident, looks him slowly up and down, and breaks the silence with two words: 'Brilliant creature'."

Along with his mentor Spence, he was one of the doctors in the Infirmary who was extremely skeptical of Lister's germ theory (unlike Joe Bell). He was not a scoffer like Spence, who would chortle in the gentle Lister's presence, "Shut the door; keep oot the germs." He suspended judgment.

Perhaps more significant than any other facet of his life to the student of detective fiction is the fact that Patrick Watson not only has a "claim" for being the original for Dr. Watson, he very well may have been, in young Conan Doyle's eyes, *the* Dr. Watson of his stories. He was a brown, mustachioed military man, trained in the Crimea. When young Doyle sat down to choose his classes at the University, he always had a choice of two instructors teaching clinical surgery: Joe Bell and Patrick Heron Watson. After one class with Dr. Bell, of course, he was hooked. Here was one area where Dr. Bell outshone his colleague, but Watson's fame as a skilled surgeon, an expert in forensic medicine, an expert on gunshot wounds, and from all accounts—a crack shot with a rifle or pistol— were well known to all the students.

The Sherlockian aficionado will say, "Yes, Yes, but what about John Dickson Carr's medical model, the James Watson of Southsea, where Conan Doyle first practised?" In an article reprinted in the *Baker Street Miscellanea* for April, 1975, "John H. Watson Never Went to China," Jay Finley Christ, one of the more scholarly Sherlockians, proves almost beyond doubt that young Conan Doyle certainly knew Dr. James Watson in Southsea, but *not* until *after* he had written *A Study in Scarlet.* Jon L. Lellenberg and W.O.B. Lofts corroborate Christ's findings. Lellenberg and Lofts, in fact, present an even stronger argument, coming up with a solid case for what Heron Watson had "most pointedly in common with John H. Watson from an auctorial point of view." Before leaving Dr. Watson of Edinburgh, we should mention two phases of his medical career that would especially interest the modern reader: he became one of Edinburgh's leading authorities on dietetics, and in 1865 published a most atypical article in the esteemed *Edinburgh Journal of Medicine* on Acupressure. Joseph Bell was mourning the death of a giant of a man—a man who was appointed Surgeon to the Queen and knighted a few years before his death.

It may have been a time of much mourning, but Joe Bell also learned to drive once he had purchased an automobile, and thus spent a good amount of time polishing his skills on the road. At the same time, it seems, he became a serious gardener, "spending as much time in the garden and the laboratory on his precious flowers as he spent on work with the blood in that same laboratory," according to Professor Caird. According to his granddaughter, Mrs. John Fulton, he was walking further than ever with her at Mauricewood; had become such an expert on ornithology and botany that bird lovers and nature lovers came calling endlessly, barraging him with questions, but he seemed to dote on the give-and-take.[130] One other curious thing, as Mr. Holmes would say, is revealed about the good doctor by Edith Fulton. While Joe Bell repeatedly told his offspring to "use your eyes, use your eyes," he himself, much like famed baseball star and expert hunter Ted Williams, would pick up a bird on the wing long before his hunting companions. The look of eagles.

On a Sunday morning in February of 1911 he made his rounds as usual, seeing "one or two patients before going to church. He made sure he looked in on the son of a handyman, a man who also drove the wagons for an undertaker's establishment." It seems he had been treating the boy at no cost for over four years. Dr. John Playfair, colleague and intimate friend recalls:

Increasing breathlessness and other distressing symptoms compelled him to give in and seek... rest in bed which his condition urgently required.... Two days later heart failure threatened, and a night of great suffering and distress followed. As a last resort a small dose of morphia was given, and the doctor made a slow but excellent recovery, in time being able to move to beautiful Mauricewood.

During all the weeks and months of his illness, never a murmur nor fretful word was heard from him, and his cheerfulness, even after a bad ... night was remarkable. I shall never forget, at the morning visit, and in response to my knock at his bedroom door, the loud and cheery come in, or come in, dear boy, so glad to see you. Then he gave me, with many humourous touches, a description of his night.

All orders and suggestions were gratefully and readily accepted and carried out with unfailing punctuality—this, too, although he was no ardent believer in the power of medicine. He realized that the best he could ever hope for would be a life of quiet invalidism. He accepted the outlook with perfect resignation and composure.... When... he began to feel the end might be drawing near, he calmly and quietly asked us what we thought his prospects of life now were, requesting us to state our opinions plainly and frankly and to keep nothing back. A strong, simple Christian faith sustained him, not only then but through some of life's severest afflictions, and enabled him with a rare and lofty courage unshrinkingly to contemplate and prepare for the inevitable.[131]

Dr. Playfair is certainly borne out by one of the most wistful and weary letters that Joe Bell wrote. Nearing seventy he wrote to an old friend: "I can thoroughly see your point about death. Yours is the Greek view. 'The sun is pleasant, and, brother, there is the wind on the heath,' and so on.... I think I would be awfully bored in a tropical Eden. As you say April has its memories, but for old folks like us what month is free from them.... Be brave and don't show anybody that you believe that this is—as it is—a weary world." He was a very tired man when he died, but he was a determined Scotsman full of faith. Providentially and fittingly, he died on Edith's birthday, October 4, of 1911.

We know from the *Times* and especially the *British Medical Journal* that his funeral was one of the largest in the history of Edinburgh. All of St. George's Free Church were there; the members of the Royal College of Surgeons and Physicians; members of the University; of the Royal Infirmary; of the Longmore (Royal) Hospital for Incurables; of the Queen Victoria's Jubilee Institute for Nurses; a detachment of Army veterans; members of the Royal Hospital for Sick Children; and his patients and the general public. *The Edinburgh Academy Chronicle* said that "By Dr. Joseph Bell's death not only has the School lost one whose whole life was an example of all that goes to make for honour and success in an arduous career, but also one who, by his high standard of citizenship, leaves his native city appreciably smaller."

Mark Twain, a contemporary of Dr. Bell, once said, in his typical Mark-Twain manner, "Live, so that when you die even the undertaker will be sorry." Dr. Douglas, who served as dresser under Bell, said there was one sight at that funeral "out to the Dean" that he would never forget in his lifetime. It was the sound of the uncontrollable wailing of a huge man, one of the undertaker's helpers, dropping huge tears into the open grave. Dr. Bell had treated his pain-wracked son free of charge for years.

XIII

Coda

Will the Real Model Rest Easy

The bones of the tired Dr. Bell should be allowed to rest with those of his ancestors, friends and colleagues in the Dean Cemetery on the western edge of his beloved Edinburgh. Less than forty years ago they were disturbed slightly by a curious tilt in the press between Adrian Conan Doyle, the author's son, and those who felt that Dr. Joe Bell was indeed the model or inspiration of the great Sherlock Holmes—notably Mr. Irving Wallace.

There are letters to and by Joe Bell's descendants; there are letters and articles by avid Sherlockians; but since most of the fury fell about the head of Mr. Wallace, most of the peculiar history will come from his pen, and the reader—Sherlockian or no—must come to his own conclusions.

The entire curious debate would be an historian's dream or "meat" for the avid biographer, but let it be said at the outset that the present biographer has no desire to denigrate or hold up anyone to ridicule. There is no gainsaying the fact that Adrian Conan Doyle jumped on his steed, raised his literary lance and rode off in all directions, but he was also fiercely proud, devoted and loyal. That his impetuosity spawned beautiful *bon mots* by others was almost inevitable; that he challenged all comers was hereditary.

The first blow fell in 1943 when Hesketh Pearson, the intrepid biographer, published an "unauthorized" biography of Sir Arthur entitled *Conan Doyle*. (Later Pearson wrote Irving Wallace to say, "Though this isn't of the least importance...you call my Life of Doyle unauthorized. Actually the Doyle family, in the person of Adrian, gave me access to private material, which I acknowledged—in the note at the beginning...."[132]) Pearson was the first to irritate Adrian Conan Doyle for his observations on Joe Bell being the model for the great detective. His treatment of Sir Arthur's involvement with spiritualism also did not endear him to the author's son.

He dashed off letters to the *London Daily Telegraph* (Oct. 10, 1943); the *London Evening Standard* (Oct. 28, 1943); the *London Times* (Oct. 28, 1943). His main thesis: "My father himself was Holmes.... There was no Watson, except that one side of his nature was like my father's." He admitted to the *Evening Standard* that "Dr. Bell... certainly helped to develop my father's powers of observation.... Dr. Budd [a fellow-student of Sir Arthur and given much space by Pearson] was for a while my father's medical partner, but he had no connection with the character of Holmes."

In the letter to the *Times* he spends more time deploring Pearson's observations about his father's absentmindedness, his 20/400 powers of observation, etc. All of this "not unnaturally, has led to a renewal of the old discussion as to whether the remarkable characteristics of Holmes were based on Dr. Bell of Edinburgh University or on the strange Dr. Budd, or merely rooted in the influence of Edgar Allen [sic] Poe."

Then an article by Adrian Conan Doyle appeared in *John O'London's Weekly* for November 5, 1943: "Conan Doyle was Sherlock Holmes." In it, young Adrian avers that he had the highest personal respect for Mr. Pearson as a friend and writer, but what did he know if "he had never met my father, and is therefore in no position to judge him in this respect." A good part of the article is given over to examples of Sir Arthur's powers of observation, although Adrian does admit his father could be forgetful.

Evidently he then also dashed off a letter to the *London Daily Telegraph*, for we find *Time* magazine for November 8, 1943, announcing that Adrian Doyle, settling once and for all the "aging argument of the prototype of Sherlock Holmes," wrote the following to the *Telegraph*: "The fact is my father himself, was Sherlock Holmes. It was true that Sir Arthur was absentminded, and often put on one brown shoe and one black, but like Sherlock Holmes the accuracy of my father's deductions was startling."

We have no indication of how Adrian felt about the continuation of the *Time* story on the Doyles: "Denis Percy Stuart Conan Doyle, brother of Adrian, announced in Los Angeles that he would soon return to England, [and] stand for election to Parliament. Denis also made his periodical report that he was still chatting with Sir Arthur from time to time."

While he was getting ready to prepare a retaliatory broadside, young Conan Doyle was alerted to an "adversary" from a new direction. The other papers followed up on the Pearson material; Adrian Conan Doyle let it be known he was unhappy; the newspapers had come to Mrs. Cecil Stisted, Joe Bell's younger daughter, who was still living at Egerton House in Kent. Adrian published a letter in the *Edinburgh Evening News* of December 4, 1943, emphasizing again that "my father himself was Sherlock Holmes.... Dr. Joseph Bell did indeed help to develop my father's immense power of observation and conclusion [sic] but it must be placed on record that these powers were indubitably innate." On December 14, 1943, Mrs. Stisted wrote to the *Evening News,* forwarding a copy of the famous letter of May 4, 1892, in which the author says that it is to you [Joe Bell]

that I owe Sherlock Holmes, etc. She concludes by
asserting that she doesn't want to get involved in any
argument of this sort.

Adrian, taking off the wraps, shot back a letter to the
Evening News on January 1, 1944, stating essentially
that Mrs. Stisted missed the point. "I do not wish to
belittle Dr. Bell," he adds, "but if the doctor had been
endowed with the power to create extraordinary gifts that
were not already innate, then the Edinburgh University
course of 1876-1881 would have produced...a spate of
incarnated Sherlock Holmes," etc.

At times young Conan Doyle's logic is hard to follow,
but these early letters to the *Evening News*, in Wallace's
words, "sounded the warring note, although with
gentlemanly and chivalric restraint, out of respect (no
doubt) to the sex and age of the enemy. It was almost the
last time that Adrian Doyle would show such public
restraint in dealing with the hosts of the Dr. Bell
camp."[133]

Still seething, apparently, about all the talk of his
father's forgetfulness, lack of observation, etc., Adrian
brought out a small book in 1945, *The True Conan
Doyle*,[134] directed against "the self-styled biographers
who wrote glibly and voluminously about Arthur Conan
Doyle without ever having known him personally and
without having access to the family documents." Wallace
felt it was aimed directly at Hesketh Pearson; and S.
Tupper Bigelow, after observing that Adrian did "not
seem to like Hesketh Pearson," added that "it seemed a
shrewd guess that Adrian wrote *The True Conan Doyle*
for the sole purpose of vilifying Pearson for writing his
Conan Doyle which he apparently had the effrontery to do
without consulting Adrian at every step."[135] Calling this
slim volume "one of the funniest I have ever read,"
Bigelow goes on to point out the logical fallacies in
Adrian's attempt to link his father's characteristics with

those of his great detective; e.g., the dust-red dressing gown and curved pipe beloved by both men. As Bigelow notes, none of the dressing gowns in the Canon was dust-red, and the curved pipe affected by Mr. Holmes was the brain-child of the illustrators.

Bigelow examines two peculiar father-son statements issued by Adrian. "I would address myself to any reader," says Adrian in *The True Conan Doyle,* "who may suffer from the delusion that a son's outlook on his parent is naturally biased. It has been my experience that the very opposite is more often true." In the preface to a book that he puffed as "the real story of my father" and "the authorized biography,"—John Dickson Carr's *Sir Arthur Conan Doyle,* Adrian says, "There is perhaps no greater fallacy than the view that a son's opinions of his father must be favorably prejudiced. More often than not, the opposite is the case..." Bigelow's reply to the filial psychologist: "If this is not 'unmitigated bleat,' it is at best 'ineffable twaddle.' "[136]

It would seem that several of Dr. Bell's former students were upset by the dispute, for we find several of them deploring the whole thing. Dr. Douglas Guthrie, not able to believe much of what he was hearing, had an extensive correspondence with Major and Mrs. Stisted of Egerton. On February 6, 1946, he sent Mrs. Stisted a letter of condolence on the death of her husband; he mentions also that he is returning the letters from Conan Doyle to Dr. Bell that she had kindly sent to him; and concludes by saying, "I think that Adrian Conan Doyle adopts a very stupid attitude, as there is no doubt the 'idea' of Sherlock Holmes came from your father, and this fact in no way [denies] that Conan Doyle, as author, worked up the idea. To say that Conan Doyle himself, and not Dr. Bell *was* Sherlock Holmes is to my mind simply silly."[137]

There was a quietus until 1948 when, in May, Irving

Wallace published a short biographical article on the
doctor in the *Saturday Review of Literature:* "The
Incredible Dr. Bell."[138] The fact that it was the lead article
and was featured on the cover probably did little to soothe
the feelings of young Conan Doyle. Wallace, the first
writer to read Mrs. Saxby's book and to get in touch with
Mrs. Cecil Bell Stisted, featured the doctor's amazing
deductive powers; repeated Sir Arthur's assertion that Dr.
Bell was truly the model for Sherlock Holmes; and quoted
several of his former students' remarks about his
uncanny powers of observation and deduction.

Wasting little time, after he was shown the article,
Adrian Conan Doyle violently denounced Mr. Wallace's
scholarship, his sensitivity, his lack of respect. It was in
this letter that the youngest son, as Wallace refers to him,
first heralded the forthcoming, definitive biography of his
father: "It will be the first genuine biography of my
father...[and] is to be published simultaneously
throughout the whole world.... This great biography
containing nothing but substantial facts, will, I believe,
be the standard reference work on my father for all time to
come...."[139]

Writing about this letter years later, Wallace
remembered he was "more amused than irritated, [but]
saw no point in heightening the conflict. I do not mean to
sound lofty, not when facing so indomitable a combatant
as Adrian Conan Doyle, Keeper of the Name.[140]" The
article was quite popular, and Wallace was encouraged to
expand and use it as the lead biography in his highly
successful and unusual first book, *The Fabulous
Originals*—biographies of the real flesh-and-blood
originals of Sherlock Holmes, Jeckyll and Hyde,
Robinson Crusoe, Poe's Marie Roget, and Henry James'
Juliana Bordereau.

Published by the prestigious firm of Longmans,
Green & Co., Ltd., the book appeared throughout Great

Britain in 1956, and was widely acclaimed there as well as in the United States and Canada. Wallace was justifiably proud of Cyril Connally's glowing review in *The Sunday Times*.[141] Connally not only found the Dr. Bell chapter "one of the three most interesting studies in this book," but went on to summarize and praise the contents: "Conan Doyle envied the effortless, eccentric superman who was also an aesthete, while he Doyle waited for patients in Portsmouth....Dr. Bell practiced deduction and astounded his students. Conan Doyle created Sherlock Holmes from him, and when the fact was known Dr. Bell began to be consulted by Scotland Yard, grew more like Holmes and claimed to solve the mystery of Jack the Ripper."

Those who commented on Adrian's reaction could not play it straight. "In Geneva," wrote Irving Wallace, "Adrian Conan Doyle read the... review, and, clearly enraged, took down his rusty lance and charged off to defend the family honor." The Marquis of Donegal, then editor of *The Sherlock Holmes Journal*, first deplored the fact that there was the Doyle-Holmes-Bell controversy; then, after flatly asserting "Let us place on record here that all Sherlockians should have Wallace's book," he notes that "The ink hardly dried on Wallace's book when Adrian—a four-minute miler when it comes to filial piety—is on *The Sunday Times'* Editor's desk with the following...," and he goes on to give portions of the reply.[142]

Adrian Conan Doyle, who would often change the thrust of his charges, did so once more. In *The Sunday Times'* letter, he excoriates Mr. Wallace for still believing "in the exploded Dr. Bell-Sherlock Holmes myth," again points out his father's powers of observation, and concludes by returning to his own Bible on the subject: "Mr. Wallace has chosen to ignore established facts, many of which are cited in John Dickson Carr's biography of Conan Doyle and will amply suffice to disprove Mr. Wallace's ingenuous effort to re-create a fairy tale."[143]

Before going into two replies to Adrian Doyle's letter, one might well ask to know what Mr. Carr did say about Dr. Bell. While eventually declaring that Conan Doyle himself indeed could serve as a model for his detective, he had noted: "If [Conan Doyle] needed a model for his detective, he need look no further than a lean figure in Edinburgh, with long white dexterous hands and a piercing eye, whose deductions startled patients as they would startle a reader in print. Yes, but Joe Bell himself sometimes blundered. Could he, Joe Bell's pupil, shut his eyes and throw himself into an artificial state of mind so that he could deduce too?"[144] That was Doyle in 1886. Carr says the following about Doyle, basking in his fame in 1892: "To interviewers who flocked to South Norwood that summer, he [Doyle] gave all the credit to Dr. Joseph Bell, whose photograph now stood on the mantlepiece in the study. Dr. Bell quickly and generously disclaimed this."[145]

Wallace, who says little about his own reply in *The Sunday Times*, accepted the challenge, and reiterated his views that the star witness for Dr. Bell as a model for Sherlock Holmes was Conan Doyle himself; he mentions the letters that Conan Doyle wrote to Dr. Bell on the same subject; and adds that he had the same evidence from many of Dr. Bell's former students, for Irving Wallace did indeed meet and correspond with several of them.

On that same Sunday Mr. J.L.H. Stisted, Joe Bell's grandson, also wrote to *The Sunday Times* from the town where the actual Battle of Hastings was fought—a town that with characteristic British understatement was named Battle. From Battle, Mr. Stisted, to use Bigelow's metaphor, "entered the lists." Mr. Stisted averred that he had five letters from Conan Doyle to his grandfather [all of them still extant] on the Dr. Bell-Sherlock Holmes argument.

The next shot, as it were, was a letter fired off to Longmans, Green & Co. by a law firm representing Adrian Conan Doyle or the Doyle family. The law firm, "fearsomely named Vertue and Churcher, Amalgamated with Gush, Phillips, Walters and Williams," in Wallace's words, "wrote that their clients were concerned about 'certain totally false and damaging statements'," in his story on Dr. Bell.[146] This time, according to Wallace, the thing that bothered the clients most was Wallace's assertion that Conan Doyle wrote Dr. Bell, asking him for more Sherlock Holmes plots and thanking him for those received. Wallace was advised to print an immediate retraction unless he could provide evidence of Conan Doyle's writing the letters. If he failed to provide evidence or an apology, the Doyle family would take action to "protect the value of their copyright and Sir Arthur's memory from fabricated writings calculated to damage it."[147] Thus Adrian (and perhaps others) had entered the legal lists. Family pride, honor and loyalty is one (or three) things, but litigation is another matter.

Irving Wallace says, "The celebrated New York copyright attorney Phillip Wittenberg" heard of his case, and told the author that in his opinion the Doyle family really had no case.

With the family waiting in the wings, Wallace wrote a letter to Longmans, Green & Co. in London, essentially telling them what Conan Doyle said in his autobiography, and that he was enclosing copies of the author's correspondence with his former mentor. Wallace never again heard from Vertue, and Churcher and Gush, et al. "I felt," he says, "I had silenced the Doyle family for all time. As before I was mistaken, for I had underestimated the wrath and energy of the youngest son.... In his Swiss retreat at 3 Quai Turrettini, Geneva, Adrian Conan Doyle was apparently contemplating his bent lance...."[148]

If he could not have Wallace in the dock he would have him in the press, and so early in 1957 Adrian began writing to just about every newspaper that would print his letters, including the *Northern Echo*, the *Bristol Evening World,* the *Bulletin* (Glasgow) and *Scots Pictorial* of Glasgow. Wallace followed all of these, and was reluctant to gird his literary loins for yet another battle, for "I felt any new defense I made would engage me, possibly unto eternity, with a seemingly tireless opponent," but he also felt that his literary integrity was at stake.

Young Conan Doyle's most detailed, most involved letter was the one that appeared in the *Northern Echo* of February 5, 1957. Wallace, to his credit, quoted it in its entirety in "What-has-happened-since" section at the end of *The Sunday Gentleman*. In it young Doyle says that he "never denied that Dr. Bell played a distinguished part in setting the model for Holmes' method in my father's mind and in developing the latter's own powers of observation." What then does bother the young man? He seems perturbed that Stevenson recognized Bell immediately as the model, but notes that in 1894 Stevenson said, "In the forefront of every battle for justice will be seen the white plume of Conan Doyle." He reminds the *Echo*'s readers that his father solved a couple of true-life mysteries; that Conan Doyle, not Bell, created Sherlock Holmes; that his father was (like white-plumed Cyrano) a champion of justice. He then complains that an expert criminologist informed him that he could find no mention of Dr. Bell's involvement in the Chantrelle case; that there is no truth that his father wrote to Dr. Bell, asking for Holmes' plots; and, finally, that "Mr. Wallace missed a golden opportunity. Had he been a researcher, he would have found himself engrossed in my father's wonderful archives...," etc. He did have one point: it is indeed difficult to learn of Dr. Bell's involvement in the

Chantrelle case.

Wallace's reply to the *Northern Echo* appeared on March 27, 1957, and he wrote to every other paper that printed young Doyle's letter. "While one must, indeed, admire Mr. Doyle's filial devotion, one cannot help but feel that this very devotion detracts from his objectivity," he began. "That is the analysis in the proverbial nutshell." Wallace then goes on to recite Sir Arthur's own admissions in his autobiography and his letters to Dr. Bell; and the corroboration of dozens of Dr. Bell's former students. Then Mr. Wallace, unfortunately, goes on to retaliate. Joe Bell too solved all kinds of true-life crimes. The irony, of course, is that neither Dr. Bell nor Conan Doyle was solving crimes when the latter was looking for a model for a detective. Wallace includes a genuinely warm paean of praise for Sir Arthur as a creative genius, and concludes: "With the publication of my letter, there came silence and peace, and it was wonderful.... This zany literary conflict about who was the real Sherlock Holmes ended in 1957, and has not been revived to this day [1965.]" How wrong he was!

Two years later (1959) Hasketh Pearson typed out a script that he would deliver on the BBC as a Conan Doyle Centenary Talk. The talk, according to Mr. Pearson and Jon Lellenberg, editor of the *Dispatch Box Press*, was cancelled by the station "when Adrian Conan Doyle threatened to deny any use of copyrighted Conan Doyle material by the BBC if Pearson was allowed to give a talk." A modified version of the talk appeared in *The Sunday Times* of May 17, 1959, entitled "More than Sherlock Holmes. Sir Arthur Conan Doyle 1859-1930." The delightful Joe Bell anecdote about the man from Liberton with the peculiar clay on his feet did not appear.[149]

Writing from Chateau de Lucens in Lucens, Switzerland, Adrian Conan Doyle wrote yet another letter—this time to the *Sherlock Holmes Journal.*[150] He begins with: "Sir—It is not my habit to break into print whenever somebody suggests that my father's creation, Sherlock Holmes, was modelled on Alice in Wonderland or Robinson Crusoe...." The editors introduce his letter with "Once more unto the Breach, dear friends."

On this occasion Mr. Doyle displayed his own brand of pawky humor. His first example is interesting: "Mr. Irving Wallace, who I believe, pounds a typewriter in Hollywood," etc. He asserts that Wallace knows little about Holmes, less about Dr. Bell, and nothing about Conan Doyle; he takes up the Chantrelle case again; and he quibbles about Wallace's assertions that Conan Doyle asked Dr. Bell for plot-ideas. The son gleefully reports that his father never made use of the plots, and quotes Dr. Bell's modest denial that he (Bell) was the model. Well, the letters asking for plots are extant, and it is certainly true that in his autobiography Conan Doyle says he did not use any of Dr. Bell's ideas, but all of this seems beside the point again. Sir Arthur was afraid to touch the germ-warfare plot and probably didn't use any other suggestions. In all fairness to Mr. Wallace he does not claim—really—that Dr. Bell's plots turned up in the Holmes stories.

Stoutly maintaining they will not take sides, the editors conclude by echoing some of Mr. Wallace's earlier language: "It is now up to Wallace to don *his* armour—*and give battle.*" Peace—it *is* wonderful.

The final thing to disturb the rest of the good doctor is rather surprising. Despite the fact that he was self-effacing, modest and shy, myths and legends did grow up around the man. Many people were convinced he headed up Bell's Scotch Distillery. The citizens of Egerton swore that he limped after a bout of sucking out poisonous snake venom. (Even Irving Wallace, who knew of his heroics during the 1864 diptheria epidemic, said he limped because of an old hunting accident.)

Cuthbert D. Smith, a sober citizen of Des Moines, Iowa, insisted that not only was his father, William Smith, the model for Dr. Watson, but also that Alexander Graham Bell was a second cousin of Sir Joseph Bell [sic], and sent the good doctor "the first telephone set ever to cross the Atlantic."[151] Sir Joseph and the author's father, a medical student in Edinburgh, rigged it up, and held "the first telephone conversation in the British Isles." Joe Bell's grandchildren should have called him "Rigs."

All in all, he was a fitting model for one of the most heroic of all literary creations. He would appeal, as Doyle said in a different context, to the boy in every man and the man in every boy. In his own day he appealed also to the little E. Winifred Binnings and most of the Victorian ladies who knew him. It seems everyone—Wallace, Bigelow and the Marquis of Donegal—end their perorations on Dr. Bell by quoting his star pupil. Who are we to differ? "So," as Jonathan Small affably asked in *The Sign of the Four,* "is there any other point you would like to ask about?"

Notes
Chapter 1

[1]Arthur Conan Doyle, *Memories and Adventures* (Boston, Little Brown & Co.), 1924, p. 69.

[2]All passages from Gaboriau are from Emile Gaboriau, *Monsieur Lecoq* (New York: Dover Publications), 1975.

Chapter 2

[3]Materials relating to the Bell family lineage and the early schooling of Joe Bell came from a private family history kept by Benjamin Bell and from newspaper accounts, especially *The Scotsman,* at the time of Joe Bell's death (October 4, 1911).

[4]Saxby, p. 53.

Chapter 3

[5]Magnusson, p. 19.

[6]*Ibid.,* p. 53.

[7]*Ibid.,* p. 84.

[8]From the original catalogs supplied by the Hon. Archivist, B.A. Stenhouse.

[9]Magnusson, p. 65.

[10]See Magnusson, p. 25, ff.

Chapter 5

[11]G.S. Stephenson, *Reminiscences of a Student's Life at Edinburgh in the Seventies.* Edinburgh: Oliver and Boyd, 1918, p. 70.

[12]Sir Robert Falconer, "In Edinburgh Fifty Years Ago," *Queens Quarterly* (November 1937), p. 445.

[13]Eric Robertson, "Student Life at Edinburgh University," *University of Edinburgh Journal* XV, No. 3 (Autumn, 1950), 673-674.

[14]*Memories and Adventures*, pp. 18-19.

[15]D.B. Horn, *A Short History of the University of Edinburgh 1556-1889.* Edinburgh: University of Edinburgh Press, 1967, p. 180.

[16]G.S. Stephenson, *Reminiscences,* p. 61.

[17]From the long obituary of Dr. Bell in *The Scotsman* for October 5, 1911.

[18]*Ibid.*

[19]Much more about Dr. Patrick Heron Watson, Dr. Bell's friend and medical luminary, will appear below.

[20]W.H. Makey, *The Society of the High Constables of Edinburgh.* Edinburgh: The Society of the High Constables of Edinburgh, 1975, pp. 3-4.

[21]Joseph Bell, "James Syme, Surgeon," in *Famous Edinburgh Students,* ed. W. Scott Stevenson. Edinburgh: T.N. Foulis, 1916.

[22]One of Dr. Brown's most famous essays on medicine.

[23]A. Logan Turner, pp. 180-181.

[24]*Ibid.,* p. 183.

[25]Much of the Burke-Hare material is drawn from that celebrated Scottish chronicler of famous trials: William Roughead, *Famous Scottish and British Trials: Burke and Hare.* London: W. Hodge, 1948.

[26]A "close" was an entry or passageway; "but" and "ben," the outer and inner rooms of most two-family dwellings in Scotland.

[27]A. Logan Turner, p. 229.

[28]*Ibid.*

[29]The Royal Hospital for Sick Children was situated at the southwest corner of George Watson's Hospital in 1869.

[30]J.S., "Lays of the Colleges" (1886). Quoted by A. Logan Turner, p. 231.

[31]The fascinating role of the Extra-Curricular teachers (of whom Joe Bell was one) and the sites will be examined when Dr. Bell and young Conan Doyle first meet.

[32]*The Scotsman,* February 20, 1960, p. 3.

[33]Operative surgery: surgery taught in the operating theatre; systematic surgery: a lecture course on the principles and practise of surgery; clinical surgery: surgery taught on the wards.

Chapter 6

[34]William Ernest Henley, *Poems.* New York: Chas. Scribner's Sons, 1898, p. 13.

[35]Saxby, p. 69.

[36]*Storming the Citadel,* p. 26.

[37]A. Logan Turner, p. 166.

Chapter 7

[38]F.H. Robarts, "The Origins of Paediatric Surgery in Edinburgh," *Journal of the Royal College of Surgeons in Edinburgh*. XIV (November, 1969), 302.

[39]C.E. Douglas, "Clinical Recollections and Reflections: Lister and his Contemporaries in Edinburgh," *Edinburgh Medical Journal*. 45 (October 1938), 810.

[40]John D. Comrie, II, 510.

[41]See especially Sir Sidney Smith, *Mostly Murder,* London: George H. Harrap & Co., 1960. Sir Sidney himself was one of the outstanding forensic experts for the Crown in this century.

[42]Saxby, pp. 18-19.

[43]"Joseph Bell," *Boston Medical and Surgical Journal*. 165 (December, 1911), 584.

Chapter 8

[44]From Henley's *Poems,* p.6.

[45]Clement Bryce Gunn, *Leaves from the Life of a Country Doctor,* ed. Rutherford Crockett. Edinburgh: Moray Press, 1935, pp. 35-36.

[46]See Irving Wallace, *The Fabulous Originals*. New York: Alfred A. Knopf, 1955, pp. 29-30.

[47]From the manuscript of a talk that was to have been delivered on the BBC by Hesketh Pearson in 1959 for the Conan Doyle Centenary. We will examine the interesting aftermath below.

[48]Dr. Harold E. Jones, "The Original of Sherlock Holmes," *Colliers*. 32, No. 15 (January 9, 1904), 14.

[49]*Memories and Adventures,* p. 26.

[50]C.E. Douglas, Obituary of Joe Bell in the *Edinburgh Medical Journal* for November, 1911. There were seven signed pieces in the obituary, following a long, unsigned, introductory obituary by the editors—ten pages altogether.

[51]Charles Edward MacGillivray, "Some Memories of Old Harveians", *Edinburgh Medical Journal* VIII (January 1912), 121. The Society was, of course, named after Sir William Harvey, discoverer of "the true course of the blood through the human body."

[52]Saxby, p. 51.

[53]Vincent Starrett, "Dr. Bell and Dr. Black," *Baker Street Journal*. VII, No. 4 (October, 1957), 197-201.

[54]*Ibid.,* 198.

[55]Lord Baden-Powell, *Scouting for Boys. A Handbook for*

Instruction in Good Citizenship. London: C.A. Pearson, 1909, p. 156.

[56]A.L. Curor, "Dr. Bell Our Teacher," *Daily Express* (London), July 11, 1930.

[57]According to Turner, 15,000 patients were seen in the Infirmary outpatient clinic in 1879-80; and each surgeon appointed from four to nine dressers every six months.

[58]Harry How, "A Day With Conan Doyle," *The Strand Magazine.* IV (August 1892), 186.

[59]From *A Treasury of Victorian Detective Stories,* ed. Everett F. Bleiler. New York: Chas. A. Scribner's, 1979, 273-285.

[60]"Recollections," p. 274.

[61]Comrie, II, 669.

[62]Douglas Guthrie, *Extra-Mural Medical Education in Edinburgh.* Edinburgh: E & S Livingstone, 1965, p. 22.

[63]The Edinburgh equivalent of London's famed Harley Street.

[64]Wallace, *The Fabulous Originals,* p. 27.

[65]Saxby, p. 87.

[66]Doyle's name was not on the list, but not because he wouldn't have been a supporter. In 1882 he was just returning from a singular adventure to Africa as a ship's doctor, and then "ran out to Plymouth" to become an assistant to an old classmate. Later in the year he started his own practice in Southsea.

[67]C.E. Douglas, "Lister and his Contemporaries," 810.

[68]*Edinburgh Academy Chronicle. XIX* (November, 1911), 29.

Chapter 9

[69]*Edinburgh Medical Journal,* XXXII, No. 12 (June 1887), 1145.

[70]*Ibid.*

[71]*Royal Hospital for Sick Children,* p. 60.

[72]This was but one of the many secret charities of the Scotsman who was supposed to cling tightly to his money.

[73]F.H. Robarts, *op. cit.,* 303.

[74]Douglas Guthrie, "Dr. Joseph Bell and Others," *Medicine Illustrated.* 3, No. 5 (May 1949), 226.

[75]In a letter from Miss Gunn to the author dated September 25, 1979.

[76]The entire account may be found in one of Conan Doyle's favorite popular magazines: "The Real Sherlock Holmes," *Tit-Bits.* LI (October 21, 1911), 127.

[77]"A Study in Terror" (1965) and "Murder by Decree" (1979).

[78]Irving Wallace, *The Sunday Gentleman.* New York: Bantam Books, 1976, p. 470. Originally published in 1965 by Simon and Schuster.

Chapter 10

[79]The letter is in the possesion of Brig. Nigel Stisted, great-grandson of Dr. Bell.

[80]Saxby, pp. 21-22

[81]*Fabulous Originals,* pp. 34-35.

[82]Henry Mills Alden, "The Original of Sherlock Holmes," *Harper's Weekly Magazine.* XXXVIII, No. 1937 (February 3, 1894), 114.

[83]Saxby, pp. 19-20.

[84]See Doyle's "The Adventures of the Six Napoleons."

[85]See *A Study in Scarlet.*

[86]See *The Valley of Fear* and "The Adventure of Thor Bridge."

[87]See "The Gloria Scott."

[88]See "The Adventure of the Greek Interpreter."

[89]See "The Gloria Scott."

[90]See *The Sign of the Four.*

[91]The gold mohur was the most common gold coin in British India; the maoris were the so-called aborigines of New Zealand.

[92]Sir Francis Galton (1822-1911), celebrated British scientist.

[93]*Fabulous Originals,* p. 35.

[94]Dr. Douglas Guthrie, "Sherlock Holmes and Medicine," from the *Canadian Medical Association Journal* (October 28, 1961), reprinted in *The Sherlock Holmes Journal.* 5, No. 4 (Spring 1962), 112-116.

[95]*Ibid.,* 113.

[96]Pierre Nordon, *Conan Doyle: A Biography.* New York: Holt Rinehart & Winston, (1967), pp. 213-214.

[97]"The Late Dr. Joseph Bell," Edinburgh Academy Chronicle. XIX (November 1911), 31.

[98]Saxby, p. 23.

[99]*Ibid.,* p. 13.

[100]Dr. Bell definitely suggested detective-fiction plots to Conan Doyle and Mrs. Saxby.

[101]Years later (1929), Dorothy Sayers made the same observation in the introduction to her anthology *The Omnibus of Crime.*

[102]*The Gamekeeper at Home* was a series of naturalistic essays by Richard Jeffries (1848-1887), an early-day British champion of Conservation.

[103]Gilbert White of Selborn (1720-1793). *His Natural History of Selborn* is the record of the bird, animal, and plant life of his native village. The book has been described as "the first to raise natural history to the level of literature."

[104]Fortune Castille du Boisgobey (1824-1891), French writer of

detective fiction.

[105]"The Flowers of the Forest," written by the Scottish poetess Jane Elliot (1727-1805), is one of the oldest and best-known dirges or ballads that laments the loss of young men's lives in battle. It is still played at funerals in Scotland, often on the bagpipe.

[106]From the obituary of Dr. Bell in *The Edinburgh Medical Journal* for October, 1911.

[107]From *The Fabulous Originals,* p. 39.

[108]*The Morning Leader* (London), December, 1893, p. 5.

[109]*Fabulous Originals,* pp. 39-40.

Chapter 11

[110]In a follow-up story (October 12, 1911), to their obituary of Joe Bell (October 5, 1911), the *Times* noted: "He was an ideal witness, cool, collected, accurate, and concise, and there were few cases, whether criminal or civil, in which his expert knowledge was not called for either by the Crown or the opposite side."

[111]*Edinburgh Evening News.* February 20, 1943, p. 5.

[112]Saxby, pp. 39-40.

[113]"Oom Paul" Kruger (1825-1904) was too old in the Boer War to lead the Transvaal forces, but he obviously still served as a bogey man.

[114]Saxby, pp. 40-41.

[115]*Theophrastus Such* was a series of essays by George Eliot (1879); the other two books are *Religious Lives* by Dean Walter Farquhar Hook, Dean of Chichester; and Samuel ("Soapy Sam") Wilberforce's *Diary and Correspondence.* The latter was the Bishop of Oxford and best known probably as an opponent of Darwin's new theories.

[116]David Daiches, "Trebblers, Bleggages, Persians," *New Yorker* XXX, 18 (June 19, 1954), 78.

[117]*Ibid.*

[118]Mr. Bengis did "pick up on" Dr. Bell's apparent flirtation with Spiritualism, a subject that will be examined below.

[119]His favorite anecdote, according to Dr. Curor, was the story of the practical Scot lad in Sunday School, who, when the Minister said, enthusiastically, "Aye, well now, what would it be like, eh, to live in a Land of Milk and Honey," answered, "Sticky, Sair. Very sticky."

[120]In a letter to the author from Agnes Watt, Secretary to the Editor of *The Scotsman,* dated February 28, 1980.

[121]C.F. Barbour, *The Life of Alexander Whyte,* p. 135.

[122]*Ibid.,* p. 136.

[123]*Ibid.,* pp. 250-251.

[124]*Ibid.*, p. 251.

[125]*Ibid.*, p. 127.

[126]Eric Linklater, *City of Enchantment, Edinburgh*, p. 134.

[127]*Fabulous Originals*, pp. 30-31.

Chapter 12

[128]John Dickson Carr, *The Life of Sir Arthur Conan Doyle*, New York: Harper, 1949, p. 44.

[129]C.E. Douglas, "Lister and his Contemporaries," 810.

[130]*The Edinburgh Evening News*, February 20, 1943, p. 5.

[131]*Edinburgh Medical Journal* 7 (October 1911), 462.

Coda

[132]*The Sunday Gentleman*, p. 476.

[133]*Ibid.*

[134]Adrian Conan Doyle, *The True Conan Doyle*. London: John Murray, 1945.

[135]S. Tupper Bigelow, "In Defense of Joseph Bell," *Baker Street Journal*. 10, No. 4 (October 1960), 210.

[136]*Ibid.*, pp. 211-212.

[137]This letter is in the possession of Brig. and Mrs. J.N. Stisted.

[138]Irving Wallace, "The Incredible Dr. Bell," *Saturday Review of Literature*, XXXI, No. 10 (May 1, 1948), 7-8, 28.

[139]In *Saturday Review of Literature*. XXXI, No. 32 (August 7, 1948), 23.

[140]*The Sunday Gentleman*, p. 477.

[141]*Ibid.*, p. 478.

[142]Marquis of Donegal, "Filial Three-Pipe Problem" *The Sherlock Holmes Journal*. 3, No. 2 (Winter 1956), 1.

[143]Letter to *The Sunday Times*, November 18, 1956, p. 8.

[144]*The Life of Sir Arthur Conan Doyle*, p. 44.

[145]*Ibid.*, p. 73.

[146]*The Sunday Gentleman*, p. 478.

[147]*Ibid.*, p. 479.

[148]*Ibid.*

[149]A noted Sherlockian sent the author a copy of Pearson's original, uncensored manuscript.

[150]*Sherlock Holmes Journal*. 7, No. 4 (Spring 1966), 130-131.

[151]Cuthbert D. Smith, "Watson's Son Reveals Real Sherlock Holmes," *Des Moines Sunday Register*. January 16, 1938 (Magazine Section), p. 2.

Bibliography

Baden-Powell, Robert. *Scouting for Boys. A Handbook for Instruction in Good Citizenship.* London: C.A. Pearson, 1909.

Barbour, G.F. *The Life of Alexander Whyte.* New York: George H. Doran Co., 1924.

Bell, E. Moberly. *Storming the Citadel: The Rise of the Woman Doctor.* London: Constable & Co., 1953.

Bell, Benjamin. *Private Family History*, n.d.

Bell, Joseph. *A Manual on the Operation of Surgery for the Use of Senior Students, House Surgeons, and Junior Practitioners.* 7th ed. Edinburgh: Oliver and Boyd, 1892.

_____ "James Syme, Surgeon," in *Famous Edinburgh Students*, ed. W. Scott Stevenson. Edinburgh: T.N. Foulis, 1916, pp. 123-131.

_____ *Notes on Surgery for Nurses.* 6th ed. New York: William Wood & Co., 1906.

_____ *Journal*, unpublished.

Carr, John Dickson. *The Life of Sir Arthur Conan Doyle.* New York: Harper and Brothers, 1949.

Christison, Robert. *The Life of Sir Robert Christison, Bart.*, ed. by his sons. 2 vols. Edinburgh: William Blackwood & Sons, 1885.

_____ *A Treatise on Poisons in Relation to Medical Jurisprudence, Physiology, and the Practise of Physic.* 2nd ed. Edinburgh: Adam Black, 1832.

Cockburn, Henry. *Memorials of His Time.* Chicago: University of Chicago Press, 1974.

Comrie, John D. *History of Scottish Medicine.* 2 vols. London: Bailliere, Tindall & Cox, 1932.

Doyle, Adrian Conan. *The True Conan Doyle.* London: John Murray, 1945.

Doyle, Arthur Conan. *The Annotated Sherlock Holmes,* ed. William S. Baring-Gould. 2 vols. New York: Clarkson N. Potter, 1967.

_____ *The Firm of Girdlestone.* London: John Murray, 1923.

_____ *Memories and Adventures.* Boston: Little, Brown & Co., 1924.

_____ "The Recollections of Captain Wilkie," reprinted in *A Treasury of Victorian Detective Stories,* ed. Everett F. Bleiler. New York: Scribners, 1979, pp. 273-285.

Gaboriau, Emile. *Monsieur Le Coq.* New York: Dover Publications, 1975.

Grant, Sir Alexander. *The Story of the University of Edinburgh.* 2 vols. London: Longmans, Green & Co., 1884.

Gray, J. *History of the Royal Medical Society,* ed. Douglas Guthrie. Edinburgh: Edinburgh University Press, 1952.

Gunn, Clement Bryce. *Leaves from the Life of a Country Doctor,* ed. Rutherford Crockett. Edinburgh: Moray Press, 1935.

Guthrie, Douglas. *Extramural Medical Education in Edinburgh and the School of Medicine of the Royal Colleges.* Edinburgh: E & S Livingstone, 1965.

_____ *Janus in the Doorway.* London: Pitman Medical Publishing Co., 1963.

_____ *Lord Lister: His Life and Doctrine.* Edinburgh: E & S Livingstone, 1949.

_____ *The Royal Edinburgh Hospital for Sick Children 1860-1960.* Edinburgh: E & S Livingstone, 1960.

Hall, Trevor H. *Sherlock Holmes and his Creator.* New York: St. Martin's Press, 1977.

Higham, Charles. *The Adventures of Conan Doyle.* New York: W.W. Norton & Co., 1976.

Horn, D.B. *A Short History of the University of Edinburgh 1556-1859.* Edinburgh: University of Edinburgh Press, 1967.

Linklater, Eric. *City of Enchantment: Edinburgh.* New York: The Macmillan Co., 1961.

Magnusson, Magnus. *The Clacken and the Slate: The Story of the Edinburgh Academy 1824-1974.* Edinburgh: Collins, 1974.

Mackey, W.H. *The Society of the High Constables of Edinburgh: A Brief History of the Society.* Edinburgh: The Society of the High Constables of Edinburgh, 1975.

More, J.W., ed. *Famous Scottish and British Trials: The Trial of A.J. Monson.* Edinburgh: W. Hodge, 1908.

Nordon, Pierre. *Conan Doyle A Biography.* New York: Holt, Rinehart & Winston, 1967.

Pearson, Hesketh. *Conan Doyle His Life and Art.* London: Methuen, 1943.

Roughead, William, ed. *Famous Scottish and British Trials: Burke and Hare.* London: W. Hodge, 1948.

Rumbelow, Donald. *The Complete Jack the Ripper.* Boston: New York Graphic Society, 1975.

Saxby, Jessie M.E. *Joseph Bell: An Appreciation by an Old Friend.* Edinburgh: Oliphant, Anderson & Ferrier, 1913.

Shepherd, John A. *Simpson and Syme of Edinburgh.* Edinburgh: E & S Livingstone, 1969.

Smith, A. Duncan, ed. *Famous Scottish and British Trials: The Trial of Eugene Chantrelle.* Edinburgh: W. Hodge, 1906.

Stephenson, G.S. *Reminiscences of a Student's Life in Edinburgh.*

Edinburgh: Oliver & Boyd, 1918.

Turner, A. Logan. *Story of a Great Hospital: The Royal Infirmary of Edinburgh 1729-1929*. Edinburgh: Oliver & Boyd, 1937.

Wallace, Irving. "The Real Sherlock Holmes," in *The Fabulous Originals*. New York: Alfred A. Knopf, 1955, pp. 22-46.

_____. "The Incredible Dr. Bell," in *The Sunday Gentleman*. New York: Bantam Books, 1976, pp. 456-485.

Major Medical Journals

British Medical Journal (1850-1911).
Edinburgh Medical and Surgical Journal (1805-1853).
Edinburgh Medical Journal (1854-1938).
The Lancet, London, (1860-1911).

Articles

Bell, Joseph. "Five Years Surgery in the Royal Hospital for Sick Children," *Edinburgh Hospital Reports,* ed. G.A. Gibson, C.W. Cathcart, D. Berry Hart, and John Thompson, I (1893), 466-474.

_____. "The Surgical Side of the Royal Infirmary of Edinburgh, 1854-1892: The Progress of a Generation," *Edinburgh Hospital Reports,* ed. G.A. Gibson, et al., I (1893), 18-34.

Bengis, Nathan L. "In Memoriam Dr. Joseph Bell," *The Sherlock Holmes Journal* 8, No. 4 (Summer 1968), 119-120.

Bigelow, S. Tupper. "In Defence of Joseph Bell," *Baker Street Journal* 10, No. 4 (October 1960), 207-212.

Chiene, John. "Looking Back: 1907-1860," *Edinburgh Medical Journal* XXII, New Series (November 1907), 410-423.

Chitnis, A.C. "Medical Education in Edinburgh, 1790-1826 and Some Victorian Social Consequences," *Medical History* 17, No. 2 (1973), 173-185.

Daiches, David. "My Father and his Father," *Commentary* XXVIII (December 1959), 522-533.

_____. "Trebblers, Bleggages, Persians," *New Yorker* XXX, 18 (June 19, 1954), 78-85.

Donegal, Marquis of. "Filial Three-Pipe Problem," *The Sherlock Holmes Journal* 3, No. 2 (Winter 1956), 1, 11.

Douglas, C.E. "Clincal Recollections and Reflections: Lister and his Contemporaries in Edinburgh," *Edinburgh Medical Journal* 45 (October 1938), 805-817.

Doyle, Arthur Conan. "Conan Doyle Tells the True Story of Sherlock Holmes," *Tit-Bits* XXXIX, No. 1000 (December 15, 1900), 287.

"Editorial Notes and News," *Edinburgh Medical Journal* VII
   (November 1911), 27.
Falconer, Sir Robert. "In Edinburgh Fifty Years Ago," *Queens
   Quarterly* XLI (Fall 1935, 441-454.
Flett, Sir John. "Memories of an Edinburgh Student 1886-1894,"
   University of Edinburgh Journal XV, No. 3 (Autumn 1950), 160-182.
Guthrie, Douglas. "Sherlock Holmes and the Medical Profession,"
   Baker Street Journal 2 (October 1947), 465-471.
____ "Sherlock Holmes and Medicine," *The Sherlock Holmes Journal* 5
   (Spring 1962), 112-116.
____ "Medicine and Detection: Dr. Joseph Bell and Others," *Medicine
   Illustrated* III, No. 5 (May 1949), 223-226
Handasyde, "The Real Sherlock Holmes," *Good Words,
   and Sunday Magazine,* (June 1902), 159-163.
Harnagel, Edward E. "Joseph Bell, M.D.—the Real Sherlock Holmes,"
   New England Journal of Medicine 258 (June 5, 1958), 1158-1159.
How, Harry. "A Day with Dr. Conan Doyle," *The Strand Magazine*
   IV (August 1892), 182-187.
Johnson, Allen S. "Doctors Afield: Arthur Conan Doyle," *New England
   Journal of Medicine* 249, No. 14 (October 1, 1953), 567-569.
Jones, Harold Emory. "The Original of Sherlock Holmes," *Collier's*
   32, No. 15 (January 9, 1904), 14-15, 20.
Kosloske, Ann M. "Sherlock Homes: Spectacular Diagnostician,"
   Marquette Medical Review 29 (January 1963), 29-31.
"The Late Dr. Joseph Bell," *Edinburgh Academy Chronicle* XIX
   (November 1911), 29-30.
MacGillivray, Charles Watson. "Some Memories of Old Harveians,"
   Edinburgh Medical Journal VIII, new series (1912), 101-122.
"The Making of the Modern Practitioner: The Passing of a Great
   Teacher," *The Hospital* 51(October 14, 1911), 45.
"The Real Sherlock Holmes," *Tit-Bits* LI (October 21, 1911), 127.
Rhynd, James. "The Man Who Sat for Sherlock," *Scots Magazine*
   (August 1930), pp. 333-336.
Robarts, F. H. "The Origins of Paediatric Surgery in Edinburgh,"
   Journal of the Royal College of Surgeons of Edinburgh XIV
   (November 1969), 299-315.
Robertson, Eric. "Student Life at Edinburgh University," *University
   of Edinburgh Journal* XV (Autumn 1950), 671-674.
Starrett, Vincent. "Dr. Bell and Dr. Black," *Baker Street Journal,* 7,
   No. 4 (October 1957), 197-203.
Wallace, Irving. "The Incredible Dr. Bell," *Saturday Review of
   Literature* XXXI, No. 18 (May 1, 1948), 7-8, 28.

Newspapers
Curor, A. L. "Dr. Bell Our Teacher," Daily Express, July 11, 1930.
Edinburgh Evening Despatch, October 9, 1911.
Edinburgh Evening News.
John, Frederick. "Was There a Real Sherlock Holmes?" *The Toledo Blade Magazine,* April 29, 1973, pp. 3, 32, 34.
"Monson's Murder Trial," *The Morning Leader* (London), December 15, 1893, p. 5.
O'Donnell, Richard W. "Elementary! Doctor Was Real Sherlock," *Boston Globe,* June 1, 1973, p. 1.
The Scotsman.
Smith, Cuthbert D. "Watson's Son Reveals Real Sherlock Holmes," *Des Moines Register,* January 16, 1938, Sunday Section, p. 2.
The Times (London), October 5, 1911, p. 9.
_____ October 12, 1911, p. 11.

Index

Bell, Laurance (Joe Bell's "sailor" brother), 214-217
Bell, Maria Isabella (Joe Bell's sister), 211
Bell, Robert (Joe Bell's brother: 1840-1912), 16
Bell, Willie ("Kinmount Willie") adventuresome ancestor of
  Joe Bell, 11
Bell and Scott, Bruce & Kerr, W.S.,
Edinburgh law firm, 18-19
Bell's Scotch Distillery, 233
Bengis, Nathan, 197-198
Bigelow, S. Tupper, 225-226, 229, 234
Binning, Mrs. E. Winnifred, 3-year-old child patient of
  Joe Bell, 164-165, 234
Black, Hugh, co-minister at St. George's Free Church,
  correspondence with Joe Bell, 136
Black, Robert K., 136
Blackethouse, 9, 12
Blackie, John Stuart, Professor of Classics, Edinburgh
  University, 42
Blackwood, Bailie, 22
Blackwood's Magazine, 21
Boer War, 196
Boisgobey, Fortune du, prolific detective fiction writer, 183
Bordereau, Juliana, 227
Boston Medical and Surgical Journal, 119
Boswell, Sir Alexander, son of James Boswell, 21
Boswell, James, 3, 20, 21, 24, 48, 51, 134
Bright, Richard, Pathologist at the University of Edinburgh,
  for whom Bright's Disease was named, 38
British Medical Journal, 211
Brown, A. Crum, Professor of Chemistry, University of
  Edinburgh, 47, 95, 101
Brown, Charlotte, 193
Brown, G.M., 212
Brown, John, doctor-author, colleague of Dr. Syme, 49, 60
Browne, Sir Thomas, 34
Browning, Robert, 9, 46, 143, 213
Budd, Dr., fellow medical student of Conan Doyle, 223
Bryce, David, Edinburgh architect, 65
Burke and Hare, 62-63
Burton, Matthew, Dr. Bell's butler, 204
Caird, Francis Mitchell, Dr. Bell's protege; Surgeon to
  the Royal Infirmary, 122, 143, 180, 219